Along the Healing Path

Recovering from Interstitial Cystitis

CATHERINE M. SIMONE

IC Hope, Ltd.
Cleveland, Ohio

Along the Healing Path
Recovering from Interstitial Cystitis

Copyright © 2000

IC Hope, Ltd.
First Printing 2000

ISBN: 978-0-9667750-1-3

Library of Congress Control Number
00-134559

Printed in the United States by:
Morris Publishing
3212 East Highway 30
Kearney, NE 68847
1-800-650-7888

This book is dedicated to someone who probably doesn't realize what a huge positive influence she has had on me, on my life, and on my healing. She not only led me to many answers along my healing path, but she did so gently and with patience. Had she not raised me to have an open mind and the courage to speak my mind, I would not be where I am today...recovered from IC. Thanks Mom, I love you!

Acknowledgements

I would like to thank God first...for all the miracles, for my healing, for my life, and especially for my husband Charlie without whom none of it would mean the same. There is really no way to thank Charlie the way he deserves to be thanked. There are no words good enough. He has been there for me through every imaginable nightmare and has never for a moment considered bailing out. His constant support and loving ways are what has kept me going through all of this. No matter what anyone thinks of me or of my writing, I always know that Charlie will love me just the same. And that's why I can do this. That's why I can write these books. It's what gives me the courage to come forward and share my thoughts with you. So if you get anything at all of value from my writing, it is Charlie you have to thank. None of it would have come to pass without him.

A special thank you to my family and to my friends. Thank you for being interested enough to take the time to read my book. Thank you for trying to understand what I went through and then for letting me know you cared. I appreciate it much more than I can express here. Your compassion and understanding has been part of my healing.

A big giant thank you to all of my IC friends, especially Barb Willis and Jane Procacci, not only for the massive support you have shown for *To Wake In Tears*, but also for the support and encouragement you gave me to continue writing. Your kindness and friendship means very much to me.

I would also like to thank all of the open minded doctors and urologists who have taken the time to not only read *To Wake In Tears*, but to call or write me with their thoughts of the book. Thank you especially for the compassion that you show to IC patients everyday.

Preface

I keep praying for confidence and inspiration as I begin writing. I keep struggling with the thought "Who am I to say? I'm just like you. I'm just another IC patient." Even as the letters and e-mails pour in with questions; always beginning with "I know you're not a doctor, but..." or "I know we're all different, but..." People just wanting to ask my opinion on what I would do in their particular situation or wondering what I think about such and such a treatment. Always they want to know, am I still doing well? Do I really believe they can get well too? Well I am, and I do. But that's only one of the many reasons I decided to write this book.

I ended up in sort of a unique position after *To Wake In Tears* was published. Yes, I had spoken to hundreds (I'm sure thousands) of IC patients over the three to four years prior to the book, but after the book came out things changed. Now I hear from even more IC patients and they are telling me about their experiences AFTER reading *To Wake In Tears*. They tell me about the changes they made in their approach to healing, the different alternative treatments they tried and how they responded. They tell me about problems they ran into and the successes that they experienced. They ask me all kinds of questions. Some I feel I can help with and others I know I can't. I have heard from IC patients who, since reading *To Wake In Tears*, have tried marshmallow root and other herbs, had their mercury fillings replaced, tried NAET, done various types of cleanses, tried the antibiotic approach, etc. I have watched as more and more people are trying alternative treatments for their IC. I have been fortunate to hear about and learn from their experiences and even more fortunate to watch as many of them begin to heal.

As I prayed for inspiration and started thinking about what I wanted to say, I began realizing that most of the people who were writing and calling me were asking me a lot of the same questions. And I started to realize that I was telling them a lot of the same things. I realized then that it would be a lot easier if I clarified certain things I said in *To Wake In Tears* and if I could offer more information on the "how to" side of things when it comes to alternative treatments and IC. First I thought, what a laugh. I was going to try to write a "how to" type book for a disease where everyone is different. Yeah...like that would be easy. But who knows, maybe if I could explain more of what I would do if I had to do it all over again, maybe it would help. And maybe if I could do a better job explaining how I did what I did and what I think about IC, especially now, looking back over my healing, who knows, maybe it might help. And maybe if I explored more of the possible "alternative" routes in recovering from IC, some that I myself have not even taken, maybe that would offer people even more options, even more hope.

I know that many of the people who will be reading this book are interested in trying the natural approach to healing their IC. Out of necessity I am speaking especially to you. I am not going to write much about the medical treatments in this book. There are plenty of sources for that information. And to understand them even more fully, please remember to ask each other about your experiences. This is very important. Other IC patients can provide you with information based on their personal experiences that doctors may not even be aware of because they haven't lived through it themselves.

In writing about the natural approach to healing IC, I wanted to make something clear. I did not turn to alternative medicine because I was angry with doctors or because I hate the medical community. (By the way, I'm not and I don't.) I turned to alternative medicine because mainstream medicine offered little hope for me to get well. It's really as simple as that. In fact, ironically enough, prior to getting IC, I was one of those people who didn't think too much of alternative medicine. My entire life my mom was into vitamins, herbs, Touch for Health (kinesiology), chiropractors, and "health foods". Because I was so healthy when I was younger and because my interests lay elsewhere, I paid little attention to what she was telling me regarding health/vitamins, etc. It's not that I thought she was "nuts" to be into all that, but I also didn't think that any of that "stuff" was going to help someone who had a serious health problem either. I thought that stuff like that was great for generally healthy people who were trying to get healthier, but certainly they were not an answer for someone who was seriously ill. I was like most people of my generation who thought that if you were sick, you go to the doctor, they give you medicine and you get better. Simple as that. And you can believe me when I tell you that I was not too pleased initially as I investigated alternative treatments for IC. It certainly wasn't my first choice for my answers to lie. I had wanted the doctors to have the answers. I had wanted *them* to fix me. And I definitely wanted it to be A LOT easier than it was. It would have been my ideal, back then, for me to find answers from modern medicine. It's really quite ironic that I am now writing a book about "alternative" ways to heal from what I consider to be a very serious illness.

Just as writing *To Wake In Tears* was part of my healing, so is the writing of this book. I have learned a lot writing this book because I decided to research even further into herbs and natural products, some things that I didn't even necessarily try myself. Those that I thought might be helpful to other IC patients, things that I would have looked into trying myself if I were still sick. I wanted to offer more options, more natural and non-invasive treatment ideas for IC patients to consider. I know now that more and more IC patients are looking for a more natural approach. I know now that there are many IC patients who have benefited from doing similar things that I did to get well. I have also noticed many people running into similar problems. I hope to expand on all of that in this book. As we all know, not every IC patient responds the same to any given treatment, whether medical or alternative. So the more options and ideas available, I think, the better. I always felt that having another treatment plan on the sidelines, waiting, just in case what I was doing wasn't working, well…it made me feel better. Instead of feeling that all my eggs were in one basket, I would always know that I had more options.

As I think of all the people out there who are still suffering with IC, my heart goes out to them. And it's difficult. It's difficult not to empathize TOO much when I speak with them or hear from them through letters and e-mails. Hearing their suffering and feeling it…because I have felt it. It's difficult to think about what they are going through, knowing their pain and suffering, knowing that I can't wave a magic wand and help them feel better RIGHT NOW. It's also difficult because as I truly wish to help people, at the same time I definitely do not wish to tell them what to do. Yes...it's difficult. The complexities and individual differences of IC make it all the more complicated. I can only hope that somehow God inspires me to offer helpful suggestions with humility, understanding always that there are as many ways to heal as there are individuals reading these words.

This book is in many ways an answer to the most common questions people ask me, especially since *To Wake In Tears* was published in November of 1998. I hope to clarify some things from my first book and to answer many of the questions that have come up since its' publication. I have included some charts and other information I hope you find helpful to refer to along your own healing path. This book is meant to be a starting point, a reference that you can go to when you're looking for ideas of things to look into further and maybe to someday try.

I hope you find something helpful among these pages.

Disclaimer

When it comes to Interstitial Cystitis and alternative treatments, which is the subject of this book, I find it difficult to say the standard disclaimer. I can't, in good conscience, tell you to just simply "check with your doctor". Instead, this disclaimer must include, check with an herbologist (a naturopath or an osteopath), check with other IC patients, and most importantly, check with yourself and check for yourself before trying any new treatment. This book is not meant to be a medical text. I am a recovered IC patient sharing my perspective and approach to healing from IC.

Introduction

If you were to read an article about IC in a magazine, you would probably read that IC is a bladder disease characterized by urinary urgency, frequency, and pain that can sometimes decrease after voiding. It might describe the fact that the bladder wall is inflamed and that some people (a small percentage they'd say) develop ulcers in their bladders. This is the typical description of IC. Only, IC is much more than that. You might even go on to read about a new drug that's out that is helping a lot of people who suffer from this mysterious bladder condition. And after reading this article, quite innocently, you probably wouldn't think of IC as that big of a deal. But you'd be wrong. Because IC, it is much more than that. If you were to ask a doctor who recognizes IC as a disease (because some still don't), you might hear from them that IC can be quite devastating for some people and they might even tell you that there are some other chronic symptoms that go along with it. They might even go so far as to say something like, "we don't know what causes it, we don't know how to cure it, but we do have ways to treat it that can make it more manageable". They would most likely tell you that they have a fairly good success rate with the treatments they offer, even though, they'd admit, different treatments work for different people. They might even imply that with a little work between doctor and patient, it's pretty reasonable to assume that they can find a way to alleviate symptoms for most people. You might think, after talking with this doctor, that IC might be awful, but at least there are treatments available. At least there are ways to live somewhat comfortably with this disease. But it's not always that easy. You see... because IC, it is much more than that.

I'd have to say, as an IC patient myself, that none of this would come close to helping a person understand what IC really is or how horrendous it can be or how there are SO many people out there still suffering terribly because there aren't any medical treatments left for them to try. Nor would they understand how many people are still undiagnosed, or misdiagnosed, or don't have a doctor knowledgeable about IC and/or willing to treat them. I'd have to say, as an IC patient myself, it is very upsetting to read these articles and talk with the doctors who seem to minimize IC, who make it seem like it's not that a big of a deal. Some articles make it seem like there is a new medication out there that is "curing" people. Now granted, this medication has helped (not cured) some people tremendously, but it's just not that easy for so many of us. The new drug only helps a very small percentage of IC patients. It is not even touted as a cure. They say it helps 38% of IC patients, which percentage-wise is not much higher than the placebo effect. Yet, when our friends and relatives read these articles in magazines or hear this from doctors, they don't know that. They don't get to see the whole picture. And I'm telling you, as an IC patient myself, that this makes life for us even more difficult. The lack of understanding of this disease is of paramount importance. Not just for research dollars (which we all know is extremely important), but also for the emotional and physical well being of IC patients everywhere. My heart breaks when I see the effects of the way the media and medical community have minimized IC. The effect that this lack of awareness is having on the individual IC patient is what I care about. It's one reason I feel it's important to speak frankly about how devastating IC can be in a person's (and in their family's) life.

IC is not just about going to the bathroom a lot, although frequency is a huge problem that prevents a decent nights sleep and disturbs or prevents many normal activities during the day. And IC is not just about having to get to the bathroom quickly (i.e., urgency) and trying to avoid an embarrassing accident. IC is about the pain. It's about having to get to the bathroom quickly or you'll be in even more pain. It's about wondering, when you get there, will you be able to go at all. It's about not knowing when you might have to be rushed to the emergency room to get catheterized. And it's about praying that whoever is on call at the emergency room when you get there has even heard of IC and doesn't think you're nuts or a drug addict. It's about feeling nauseated because you're in so much pain that its making you sick, especially when you're bladder is full. It's about having a deep, burning pain that pain medications barely touch. It's about sharp, shooting pains and dull aching pain 24 hours a day for many of us. And it's about the constant discomfort on top of that pain. IC is about having all kinds of other strange symptoms besides bladder symptoms. It's about feeling as if your body is falling apart and that there is just one thing wrong after another. It's about not knowing how you're going to feel from one minute to the next and no longer being able to make plans like a normal person. It's about not feeling like yourself anymore and not being able to do the things you used to do. It's about being left out of things because you're not well enough to attend. And then it's about dealing with family and friends who don't understand how you could be "not well enough to attend". IC is about having an invisible disease. It's about having pain that no one can see and symptoms that no one understands. It's about having family and friends look at you like you're a hypochondriac or a wimp. It's about being told you're crazy when you're totally and completely sane. No… IC is not about having to go the bathroom a lot. IC, it is MUCH more than that.

As fate would have it, I write again, beholden to no one. There is no organization, company, or group that tells me what I can or cannot say. I write and say what I believe to be true from my perspective, which is really all anyone can do. I do this with one goal in mind and that is to try and help my fellow IC patients to find relief from their suffering. My gift to you has always been my honesty and candidness about IC and I won't stop offering that now.

I write to empower others who are suffering, as I was, with a disease called Interstitial Cystitis. I choose always to give people the benefit of the doubt that they can think for themselves, decide for themselves, and know what is best for them. As you probably already know, I am not a doctor, nurse, or "healthcare provider". But I am a healer of sorts. We are all healers really. We all have the ability to heal ourselves and we all have the ability to help others heal. My books and my work on line are my effort to help others heal; to help them find their way to their own healing. This book is a patient's perspective, a patient's experience, a patient's wisdom, and a patient's research. Not only am I a patient, I am only one patient. I remind you always to look to, listen to, and talk with each other. You will always learn a lot with an open mind to others experiences, especially where IC and IC treatments are concerned.

Just because I am writing this book, does not mean that I have all the answers. I want that to be clear right up front. And, in reality, it is truly not for me to have all the answers. It is better that you find your own answers. As I always say, look to your own body and your own situation because that's where you will find the answers that are right for you. Learn as much as you can about something and then listen to your gut. Your gut instincts, your higher self, whatever you prefer to call it, it will not let you down. You can believe me when I say to you that my way is clearly NOT the only way. I hope this came through loud and clear in *To Wake In Tears*. My hope is that by reading my books and then exploring further, you will come to realize that you can find your own way. Just seeing that someone like me, an ordinary person with IC, a person just like you, can find a way, can get better, I hope will allow you to believe that you too can find a way, that you too can get better.

Again I write with that feeling. I don't want to let you down. Somehow I've been given this gift, this opportunity to talk with you and share with you how I got well. To hopefully help you find a way to get well too. I have decided again to just say how I truly feel. To say what I would say if I were sitting and talking with you in person. Things I might worry to say in a book. But I fear, that's what most people do and often the truth is brushed over, made more "suitable" for reading (and for not getting sued). But because my concern lies with you not feeling any more pain and suffering than you already have had to, there are things I feel I must say. There are things I feel are important truths to be said. You might not agree with all of my truths because we all have our own perspectives and opinions, but I do feel quite certain that some of them will be hard to disagree with. Not because they are my opinions and I think I know what I'm talking about or anything, but because the truth just has a way of doing that.

With this kind of book, out of necessity I write as though you are looking to take a similar approach to treating your IC as I took myself. I wasn't sure there would be this much interest in the way I did it as there has turned out to be. I didn't realize that this many people would be open to trying alternative treatments. But I was wrong. More and more people are looking for alternatives. One reason, I believe, is because the medical treatments available at this time are simply not working out too well for many IC patients. I am not saying this to criticize the medical community, but rather to simply state a fact. I do not begrudge anyone his or her own opinion or treatment choice where IC is concerned. We are all so different and my IC may not be the same as your IC. Not everyone who reads this book will have IC the same way I had IC. And not everyone has a severe case, thank God. Some have a moderate and some have a mild case. Read this book then, with your type of IC in mind.

I worry so much for my IC friends. I watch as they try various things to get well. I watch as they take medications and undergo procedures and "listen to their doctor". I watch as they go to the health food stores and to alternative health practitioners and I am afraid for them. Oh...I understand *why* they are doing what they are doing. And I most certainly understand their fears and worries because I have been there myself. Yet, there are so many warnings I want to scream out. Sometimes it takes everything out of me not to scream them out. But with every fiber of my being, I know and understand that everyone has to make their own way, find their own healing path, to find what works for them. I can't tell you what to do in this book. I can't tell you exactly what to do to heal from IC. But I can tell you what I did and what my opinions are based on my successes and my failures, based also on the successes and failures of other IC patients that I speak with regularly. Hopefully I can provide you with more ideas to either agree with or disagree with. Sometimes in reading something that you disagree with, it makes you even more certain; more resolved in what you know to be true for you. And in this way, if my opinions can help you then I will be very pleased. And if you do happen to agree with my views of IC and my approach to healing IC and if you would like to try to find similar ways to heal yourself, I hope very much that this book offers you many ideas and possible options to try out. But do not just listen to me. Do not do what I did just because it worked for me. Do what you think will work for you, in your situation, based on your body. The best advice I can ever offer my IC friends is to tell them to do what feels right to them. I say it so often in answer to their questions that they probably want to strangle me. I try to listen and tell them what I would do in their situation (given my perspective of IC) and then I let it go for them to decide. I will remind you again. We are all different. What works for one IC patient is not necessarily going to work for another. Take from this book then what feels right to you, and for you, and leave the rest behind.

Contents

Section 1 – A Healing Path   1

Section 2 – Steps Along the Path   31

Section 3 – Stones Along the Path   65

Section 4 – Herbs and IC   87

Section 5 – Other Natural Products   115

Section 6 – Charts and Things   141

Section 7 – Key Things to Remember   165

Endnotes and References   173

Appendix – Candida Questionnaire   179

"If I have the belief that I can do it,
I shall surely acquire the capacity to do it,
even if I may not have it at the beginning."
- Mahatma Gandhi

Section 1

---◆---

A Healing Path

I know everyone says there is no cure for IC. I realize they say there is only remission, not recovery. And in one sense, this is true. There is no known medical cure for IC. There is no procedure, no magic pill, and no single treatment that exists (yet) that is said to be a cure. There ARE procedures, pills, and treatments though. It's just that they only work for some people, and when they do work, they are usually only temporary and often incomplete. Often the pills must be taken forever (e.g., Elmiron, anti-depressants, low dose antibiotics) and/or the treatments and procedures must be repeated again and again. Sometimes treatments that used to work, stop working, and the person must try another one. Other times the side effects from the medication actually require yet another medication. I just spoke with an IC patient this afternoon that was actually told by her doctor that there is no way to stop the progression of this disease. Obviously, I completely disagree. I do believe there is recovery from Interstitial Cystitis, as well as its related chronic illnesses. I believe it not only because it has happened for me, but also because it has happened for other people that I know who have also taken a more natural, holistic approach to healing. This book is my attempt to show you how to do the same.

It's been well over a year since *To Wake In Tears* came out and I still have basically the same views of IC as I had when I finished writing it. If anything, my beliefs and opinions of what IC is (at least for many of us) have grown stronger. After what I have seen since the book came out, I am even more certain of my beliefs. As I have watched more and

1

more people try using marshmallow root tea, for example, I am more certain than ever that it's a great herb for IC patients. In other words, it wasn't just me that it helped. It is helping countless IC patients now. Watching people take a similar approach to their healing as I took has only confirmed to me what I believe IC to be. It is not that *everything* I did, they are doing. And it's not that they are doing things exactly the same way I did, but the approach, in general, is the same. Some of the variables, the most important ones, are the same. They are the ones I am about to share with you here in this book.

I will try to be brief with the intro stuff because I know that if I were in your shoes right now I would want me to get right to it. I would be looking for ideas to help me RIGHT NOW. I decided to forgo the quick summary of what happened to me, what I did to get better, and how I came to figure this all out. I told that story already in *To Wake In Tears* and aside from the great possibility that you're sick of hearing about me, I thought it might be more productive to just pick up where I left off. However, I do need to share my perspective of IC first, not only because the rest of my advice is based on my perspective, but also because not everyone reading this book will have read the other.

My perspective of IC may not be the same as yours and that is perfectly okay. This is just how I view IC and how I treated it to get well. I realize this is not the "popular" view of IC. It's not what the doctors are telling their patients and it's not what is written about in medical journals (well not yet anyway)(I'm kidding). There are tons of theories out there about the cause of IC. Some would even say that we don't all have the same IC. There really isn't much agreement yet in the medical community when it comes to this disease. There are still great debates as to whether IC is caused by an as of yet unidentified bacteria or not. There are people who feel very strongly that IC is an autoimmune disease and some who think IC is a symptom of a greater illness or syndrome. Some people believe that IC is connected to back problems and others feel certain that hormones are involved. It can get very confusing because we don't all have the same symptoms, we don't all "get" IC the same way, and we don't all respond to the same treatments. So who is right? Could it possibly be all of them?

There are so many questions. What is IC? Why are we all so different? And why do different treatments work for different people? First let me say that among all of our differences there actually are some similarities. One of those similarities, naturally, is that we all have SOME bladder symptoms. Yet, even those are not the same. Some have frequency and urgency, with no pain. Some have only pain and pressure, no frequency and no urgency. Some have urgency and pain, but their frequency isn't too bad. Okay, you get the idea. So even among our most common symptom (the bladder), we have many variations. Another similarity is that most of us have other symptoms and/or illnesses that go along with our bladder symptoms. It wasn't just me who developed all kinds of other weird symptoms when I got IC. There are many of us who have some combination of these other symptoms. I think maybe because the onset of my IC was so dramatic and so severe, that it was easier for me to recognize the connection. I think that when people develop IC more gradually, it can be more difficult to see the connection between the various symptoms. And then to add to the confusion, many people are sent to various specialists who each run their own tests and offer a label/name for each symptom. This makes it seem like they are all different diseases instead of all being a part of the same thing. Or I should say, rather than that they are all connected. You will probably not have ALL of the following symptoms yourself (well hopefully not), but please don't think you're alone in having many of them (I did) or even any of them for that matter. (By the way, this is the same list of symptoms I wrote in *To Wake In Tears*. Unfortunately, the symptoms haven't changed much.)

Bladder - Pain in the bladder that intensifies as the bladder fills and sometimes lessens upon voiding (for some), bladder pain immediately following urination, mild to extreme urgency, mild to extreme frequency (up to 85 or 100 times a day in severe cases), inability to start the urine stream, burning pain, burning during urination, cramping with sharp or shooting pains, urethra pain, blood in urine, mucous in urine, dark and/or cloudy urine, small pieces of tissue with blood attached visible in urine, bubbles in the urine, strong odor to the urine, recurrent "standard" bladder infections or urinary tract infections (UTI's), incontinence, reduced bladder capacity

Kidneys - recurring kidney infections, kidney inflammation and flank pain, burning pain and soreness in the kidneys, recurring kidney stones

Teeth - infections of the teeth and gums, mouth sores, canker sores, (a common site is the corners of the mouth), TMJ and/or jaw pain, sore tongue, burning tongue

Allergies - food and environmental allergies, sensitivity to medications (synthetic and natural), extreme chemical sensitivities

Digestive problems - acid stomach, (sometimes stomach ulcers or acid reflux), diarrhea and/or constipation, or one or the other, pain during bowel movements (Irritable Bowel Syndrome)

Nausea (increased when urine is held too long)

Pain, redness, swelling, itching, and severe irritation of the tissues covering the vaginal or vulva area (Vulvodynia)

Recurrent vaginal yeast infections and/or thrush (Candida)

Muscular and skeletal system problems - pain in all muscles and joints (Fibromyalgia)

Earaches, sore throats, sinus infections or sinus problems, lung congestion

Low-grade fevers every day

Low blood pressure (though some have high blood pressure)

Swollen glands all over the body (especially top of legs in groin area, throughout the neck and chest, and under arms)

Inflamed spleen and liver

Pain at the base of the neck

Itching with no rash present

Very accentuated PMS symptom...extreme bloating, extremely painful cramps, heavy bleeding (blood clots), irregular cycle. (All IC symptoms increase around menstrual cycle)

Migraines and/or severe headaches
Hypothyroidism (though some have hyperthyroidism)
Dry skin, dry hair, dry mouth, dry eyes (Sjogren's Syndrome)
Nerve pain down back of legs and/or arms
Bloating in pelvic area (e.g., looking like you're three months pregnant) and/or edema (swelling all over the body)
Inability to lie on left side (or right side) hip and leg
Night sweats and/or lack of perspiration
Unable to have anything touching pelvic area (clothes) due to pain
Sensitivity to bright light (painful to eyes)
Cold hands and feet (nose and ears) (Raynaud's Phenomenon)
Inability to tolerate extreme temperature changes
"Catching everything that's going around" (lowered immune system)
Lower back pain (can shoot up into the kidneys and/or down into the thighs)

Associated Illnesses (Many IC patients are also diagnosed with the following, the first four being extremely common.)
Fibromyalgia
Irritable Bowel Syndrome
Vulvodynia
Systemic candida infection
Sjogren's Syndrome
Raynauds Phenomenon
Migraines
Anemia
Mitral Valve Prolapse (MVP)
Endometriosis/cysts/fibroids
Chronic Fatigue (and Immune Deficiency) Syndrome
Systemic Lupus Erythematosus

I do think more and more people are realizing that there is a connection among their various symptoms and illnesses. Even the research is now beginning to reflect this knowledge. And though there are still doctors, who everyday continue to tell IC patients that their other "weird" symptoms are not related to their bladder, there are many who are learning that they most certainly are. As I've said before, I believe that, for the most part, the medical community has been treating IC as if the bladder were not attached to the rest of the body. Evidence of this lies in the fact that urologists are still the ones treating IC and also in the fact that the majority of treatments are aimed at the bladder and for the most part, ignore the rest of the body.

IC is not just a bladder disease.

I strongly believe that IC affects the whole body and that the whole body must be treated in order to get well. Yes, sometimes you can get into remissions by treating only your bladder. And yes, sometimes you can cover up symptoms with medications. But in my opinion, if you don't get to the source of the problem and treat your whole body, it is very difficult to get well and to stay well. And if you don't recognize or "see" the source of the problem, then possibly, what you are doing might be hurting, rather than helping, your body to heal. I have to be honest. I don't think the medical community is "seeing" IC. I think they are missing what the root of the problem is because it is simply something that they don't normally look at. It is something that certainly urologists aren't going to look at because their specialty, their main focus, is the bladder. So on to the million-dollar question...what is at the root of the problem? And how can it be the same for most IC patients if we are all so different?

I believe that our differences arise out of our one major commonality, which in my opinion is this...

IC patients have a toxic body.

We are all toxic for different reasons and to different degrees, but I have found that IC patients have pretty much the epitome of the toxic body. The more severe the IC, the more toxic and sick the rest of the body. IC patients often feel as if they are full of poison or on chemical overload. There is a feeling of too much acid in the system. (This is why antacids, baking soda and water, Prelief, and Tummy Tamers are so helpful to many IC patients. They allow them to be able to eat and drink things they normally couldn't tolerate, providing them some relief from the pain and burning.) The stomach, the intestines, the kidneys and bladder are all burning with acid. This is what IC felt like to me and to many other IC patients I've spoken to. (Some of us have joked that we should glow in the dark with how toxic we feel.) The more severe the IC, the more likely it is that the IC patient feels this way.

Evidence of our toxicity lays in many of our common symptoms. Every single part of our body that processes and eliminates toxins, is, or can be, affected with IC. The liver, spleen, lymph glands, intestines, kidneys and bladder can all be inflamed, irritated, and overworked. Problems with all the mucous membranes in the body can, and usually do, occur. From the mouth and sinuses, to the stomach and intestines, and obviously the bladder. In fact, the inflamed and irritated mucous membranes, both in the bladder and elsewhere, with typically no apparent signs of infection present, represent a classic sign; a red flag, so to speak, of a toxic body. More evidence of our toxicity lays in these other fairly common IC-related symptoms: digestive system problems (e.g., Irritable Bowel Syndrome, acid-reflux, nausea, etc.), chemical sensitivities and allergies, unexplained nerve pain and/or numbness in various parts of the body, unexplained itching with no rash present, dry eyes, mouth, skin and hair, dry everything, unexplained bloating, prone to all types of infections (bacteria, fungus, viruses) with a lowered immune system, mysterious muscle and joint pain.

I'm not saying that bacteria are not involved in IC or that candida is not involved. I'm not saying that hormones are not to blame, nor am I saying that there isn't a dysfunction occurring in the lining of the bladder in IC patients. I'm not saying that IC is not an autoimmune disease, nor am I saying that IC can't be related to back injuries or to stress. What I am saying is that ALL of this is true. All of these things can be the case for someone with IC. And what is underlying all of these things, in my opinion, is a toxic environment within the body, as

7

well as a deficiency in certain key vitamins and minerals. What is underlying all of these things is what we have in common. Unfortunately, what is underlying all of these things is also what makes IC not only totally confusing, but also allusive to mainstream medicine who is not looking in this direction. I realize that it's a bold step for me to claim to know what is at the basis, at the root cause, of IC. Some people, I'm guessing, will be horrified that I am saying this and/or will claim this not to be the case. But that's okay. I'm not writing this book to convince you or anyone else that IC patients have a toxic body. This is simply what I believe to be the case. It's what my experience with IC was all about. Looking at it this way and treating it this way is how I got better.

So what produces all these toxins? In other words, why are we so toxic? How did we get this way? First of all, there are so many sources of toxins that exist today in our "modern" society that it's astounding. We are exposed to toxins in our foods (e.g., food colorings and chemical additives, preservatives, artificial sweeteners, hormones, antibiotics, and pesticides), in our water (e.g., lead, arsenic, chlorine), in our air (e.g., exhaust fumes, perfume, cigarette smoke), and in our environment in general (e.g., chemical cleaners, carpet fibers, fertilizers). The list gets completely out of control. Until I became chemically sensitive with my IC, I had no concept of the barrage of toxins that we take on daily. We get so used to it that we don't even think about it. At least, when I was healthy, I never did. From the detergents and chemicals we use to clean our homes, and ourselves, to the exhaust fumes, cigarette smoke, and perfumes in public. And then, a lot of the food we eat has had all the natural goodness removed and replaced with chemical substitutes. Between the food colorings, preservatives, and additives, not to mention the hormones, antibiotics, and fertilizers, it's astounding that we get any nutrition at all from our foods anymore. According to the book *Well Body, Well Earth* by Michael Samuels and Hal Bennett, the average American consumes about 14 pounds of food additives per year, along with one gallon of pesticides. Approximately 2,800 additives are intentionally added to the food we eat. As many as 10,000 more additives or toxins find their way into our food indirectly as it is grown, processed, packaged, and stored. (It's enough to make you never want to eat again!) Yet, most people eat this "junk" food and most people are exposed to all of these toxins everyday, yet obviously not all of them get sick. Why is that? Among the many reasons are the ways in which the individual takes care of him or herself (e.g., diet, exercise, enough rest), the degree to which they are exposed to internal and external toxins, hereditary weaknesses, and the level of stress the person is under. How many toxins are going into the body and how many are being processed out through exercise and a healthy colon for example all plays a role. The more stressed the body is with external sources of toxins, as well as internal sources of toxins (e.g., constipation, candida), the more likely the body is to get sick.

Toxicity has increasingly been identified as a predisposing factor in all kinds of acute and chronic illnesses. From environmental illness and chronic fatigue to degenerative diseases such as MS and Alzheimers. There are so many new chronic illnesses and the amount of people getting them is increasing everyday. These chronic illnesses have many things in common and many of us who have one, seem to have more than one. Also the people who are getting these chronic illnesses are getting younger and younger. IC is an example of a chronic illness once thought to be present in mostly older women and now many of those diagnosed are in their 20's, 30's, and 40's. Even teenagers and children are getting IC. Not only are young women, teens, and children, but also more and more men are being diagnosed with IC as well.

We live in a very toxic world. We have chemicals and toxins today that did not even exist 30 years ago. We have medications and synthetic products, surgeries and "procedures" that had not been invented yet. We couldn't possibly know the extent to which all these chemicals, drugs, genetically altered foods, etc. are affecting us. Not to mention how they are affecting us all mixed together. Also of great significance, in my opinion, is that they increased the amount of mercury used in amalgam fillings back in the 1970's, which strangely enough coincides

9

with the increase in many of these mysterious chronic illnesses. I don't find it surprising that many more people my age (I'm 36 at the time of this writing) who were children in the 1970's are coming down with these mysterious chronic illnesses. Most of these newer chronic illnesses have no scientifically understood "cause" and have no "cure" either. IC, of course, is no exception.

As I said earlier, I believe that we all become toxic for different reasons. We all have different sources that got us to this point, to the point where our IC symptoms began and to the point where we are right now. For some people it might have been a combination of stress, food allergies, and smoking. For some it may have been years of taking repeated antibiotics and/or birth control pills that resulted in a yeast imbalance in their body. Some people are exposed to environmental toxins at their job on a regular basis. Some people smoke cigarettes or are consistently around others who do. Some are on prescription medications for years and never consider that they are sources of chemical toxins to their body. Some of us have consumed large quantities of diet soda and "fat-free" foods that are loaded with chemicals. Many of us have mercury amalgam fillings (or root canals and crowns that contain mercury) and we are being negatively effected by them. We are not taught that we need to protect ourselves from these things (well...smoking maybe, but not the others) or that we need to cleanse them out of our body every once in a while. If the input of toxins is much greater than the output, toxins will be stored within the body and eventually things will break down. It will not breakdown in exactly the same way for everyone.

As I mentioned earlier, not all of us get IC the same way. Some people develop IC after repeated bladder infections, some after one huge bladder infection, and some immediately following some type of abdominal or "female" surgery. Even dental surgery/dental work and car accidents have been found at the onset of IC for some people. Some people are first diagnosed with Irritable Bowel Syndrome or Fibromyalgia (or have symptoms of them) and then IC gets added to their list of mysterious chronic illnesses. Some people feel that they were born with IC or have had IC symptoms since childhood. There are others who have no idea how their IC started, it seems that they just woke up one day with IC. But if you look at what many of us have in common in terms of how we got IC, shockingly enough you can actually find some similarities.

One thing that is fairly common is that many of us were under a lot of emotional stress and/or physical stress in the form of infection or surgery for example at the onset of our IC. I also think what occurs for many people is that there is simply a breaking point. A time when the body is so out of balance, so toxic and/or stressed, that IC appears to come on suddenly. It appears to come out of the blue, but in reality, there was maybe some type of trigger…a "straw that broke the camel's back" so to speak. It can be a huge trigger like surgery or a massive infection or maybe a more subtle trigger like a lack of key nutrients in the body, an abundance of stress, or whatever, and it just took the body right over the edge. It was simply too much. The body becomes overwhelmed and reacts with symptoms. I believe the trigger can also be an allergic reaction for some people. Something that we might be allergic to and maybe we had no idea we were allergic to. Two great examples are sulfa antibiotics and latex catheters. But it can also be chlorine from a pool or hot tub or even something we've eaten. We get exposed and symptoms begin. We seem to never "bounce back".

I've found that even when it appears that IC came on dramatically, it could have been coming on for a while but maybe we just didn't realize it. I think this was the case with me. It appeared that my IC began immediately following surgery for a ruptured ovarian cyst and in many ways it did. Yet, now that I am better, looking back, I can see what happened more clearly. I can see how I was primed and ready for IC. I can see how my body was all set to get it. At the time of the surgery, my body had been severely physically stressed for two and half weeks with the poison of the ruptured cyst sitting in my abdominal cavity. I had been in so much pain during that time that I got very little sleep and I'm certain I was deficient in tons of vitamins and minerals by the time I had the surgery.

11

Looking back even further, I can also see how I was having the beginning signs of IC back in college. I never realized it at the time. I didn't even realize it as I wrote *To Wake In Tears*, but now I can see it. Now I can see where the toxins were coming from for me and how I gradually became more and more toxic over time. I realize now that I did have some symptoms back then, but I just thought they were "normal". I had always been so healthy that when I first starting having symptoms, I never even thought of them as symptoms. I started to develop mild seasonal allergies in college. The college doctor told me that it's "normal" for girls my age (I was 20) to develop allergies because our bodies are changing. I thought nothing of it. I was going to the bathroom more often than I did when I was a kid, but I just thought I was a normal female. I never had a bladder infection or anything. I thought that girls just went to the bathroom more often than guys. Back in college was the first time I ever got cramps with my period, the first time I ever had a cyst on my ovary, the first time I ever had a yeast infection, and the first time I started getting sick more easily (like with colds or flu). Again, I brushed it off thinking that this was normal for a girl my age and for a college student who was probably not eating right or taking as good care of herself as she did when she was at home. I was put on birth control pills to help stop cysts from developing and to help with the cramps and PMS symptoms. I thought nothing of taking them. Nearly every girl I knew was on them and I was told how safe they were, etc. I was given antibiotics for ear infections and chest colds and again, I thought nothing of it. I had never heard of acidophilus or intestinal flora. I had no idea antibiotics killed good bacteria along with the bad. And I certainly didn't realize that antibiotics could cause yeast infections or suppress the immune system. I was acting like most people of my generation and the generation before me, I was just "listening to my doctor". Taking his advice, because he was the expert, and then thinking nothing more of it.

So what happened to me in college when this all started? Well, as I mentioned in *To Wake In Tears*, I was accidentally hit in the face with a baseball bat that broke while we were playing softball. Several of my teeth broke, including a couple molars with big fillings in them. The dentist told me that the fillings might actually have been holding the teeth together, so we left them alone. You might remember that this was the reason why I thought I was more sensitive to the mercury in my silver fillings. A couple years ago while writing the other book, I simply thought that this injury just provided me with a weakness. I didn't realize it was necessarily the beginning of all my health problems.

Looking back even further, I also remembered back in junior high and high school (back when I was first having cavities filled) that I had a lot of stomach problems. As time went on I just took antacids and again didn't think that much of it. I mean, in college pretty much everyone is taking antacids, Alka Seltzer, Pepto Bismol or whatever. Heck our whole society takes that stuff! It took me a long time to finally figure out that mercury amalgam fillings were a major source of toxins to my body. I found that the links between mercury poisoning and my IC were huge. It will not be this way for everyone. Not everyone even has mercury fillings, but for me, it was definitely one of the major sources of toxins to my body. There were others for me as well. Cigarette smoking was major for me also. So was poor eating habits, lack of exercise, and lots and lots of emotional stress, along with the physical stress then of the ruptured cyst and surgeries.

Though it is fairly common that many of us were under a lot of stress at the onset of our IC, I do find this to be a touchy subject. And yet it's important to mention and I'll explain why. It's touchy because so often we are told that IC is in our head or that we are somehow at fault for getting IC, as if we caused ourselves to get it somehow. Obviously, I don't think that is the case. IC is VERY much a physical disease. IT IS NOT YOUR FAULT YOU HAVE IC! (Sorry didn't mean to scream.) It's so sad to me that people, for years, have been blamed for "creating" their bladder symptoms as if they were "hysterical" females or neurotic women with neurotic bladders. IC patients have been shoved over to the psychiatrists' office in way too many cases instead of being treated for a physical disease. Because of this, the idea that stress plays any role in our getting IC becomes somewhat of a touchy subject. But stress is a major factor in the body's ability to ward off illness. Stress, not only in and of itself produces toxins in the body, but stress also depletes the body of certain much-needed vitamins and minerals. Physical stress on the body can range from infection (perhaps a bladder infection, but not necessarily), allergies, and surgery, to lack of sleep and proper nutrition. Or I should say properly absorbed nutrition, because you can eat "right" and even be taking supplements, but if you're body is not absorbing the nutrition, then you're not getting the vitamins and minerals you need.

The Stress Connection

Stress does not cause IC, but stress does play a significant role in several ways. 1) Most IC patients feel that their symptoms are worse when they are under stress, (Actually, I'm not sure I've ever spoken to an IC patient who didn't feel that way.) 2) Many of us were experiencing a lot of stress at the onset of our IC symptoms (either physical or emotional stress, or both), and 3) stress is known to lower the immune system and deplete our body of certain vitamins and minerals. This is all not to mention that just having IC is very stressful. It can be very stressful before being diagnosed, when you're scared because you don't know what's wrong with you and neither does anyone else. It is especially scary for those with more severe IC. We are often petrified that we have some deadly disease because the pain is so bad and because we're bleeding from a place that we're NOT supposed to be bleeding from. During that time, prior to diagnosis, many of us are mistreated, misdiagnosed, sent to psychiatrists, or generally treated as if the pain and symptoms were in our head. (Unfortunately, this still occurs fairly often, as many doctors are still misinformed or uninformed about IC.) As many of you know, it is VERY STRESSFUL to be treated as if you're crazy when you're perfectly sane and really very sick. Then, even after finally being diagnosed, IC remains a stressful disease for many of us. Among other things, we stress about each new scary symptom that occurs, we stress about where and when we can find the next bathroom and whether we will make it there in time, we stress about our friends and family not understanding what's wrong with us, we stress about whether we will be able to make it to things like family holiday celebrations, and on top of all that and more, we stress about the fact that there is no cure. And during all this time, we endure the physical stress of being sick to begin with.

When I was sick with IC, I always got much worse symptom-wise during any and all stressful situations. Pain and tingling would go down the backs of my arms and down into my pinky fingers which would go numb, my bladder would spasm and stop working, sometimes my IBS symptoms would kick in, I'd feel nauseated and a million times worse in every way. Once the stressful situation passed, I would still have to deal with the physical aftermath for hours and often the rest of the day. It amazed me how the release of adrenaline or whatever it was that happened when I would get really upset, angry, stressed out, etc. had on my IC symptoms and my entire body. There was no question about it. When I was sick with IC, any and all stress made me MUCH worse. If you have a moderate to mild case of IC, your symptoms during stress might not be as dramatic, but you probably can still tell that it's negatively affecting you, even if it's just an increase in frequency.

Stress, whether physical or emotional, depletes certain vitamins and minerals in the body, as well as lowers the immune system. All types of stress, including emotional stress, deplete the body of B vitamins. **Another thing that I believe many (dare I say nearly all) IC patients have in common is a tremendous deficiency in the B complex vitamins.**

Not only are we extremely deficient in the B vitamins, most of us cannot tolerate taking them either. Not only do supplements containing B vitamins cause burning pain for most IC patients, but also foods that contain B vitamins can also cause burning. The B complex vitamins are absolutely crucial to our body's ability to handle stress, not to mention a multitude of other bodily processes. I really think this is one of the major reasons why IC patients have such trouble with anxiety and some even suffer panic attacks. I also think it's one of the reasons why stress brings on "flares" for many people and why IC patients have more trouble *physically* dealing with stress and anxiety. Often we blame ourselves (I say often, but what I really mean is nearly all the time), but I strongly believe that it is a nutritional deficiency that is to blame, NOT our "mental and emotional capabilities". Along with a toxic body, a serious deficiency in the B complex vitamins, in my opinion, is another VERY important common thread among IC patients.

There are other vitamin and mineral deficiencies common among IC patients that are not only intimately linked with the organs/body systems that we most often have problems with, but are often ignored as playing any role at all in the person being ill. It is recognized that we can't tolerate certain vitamin supplements (e.g., Vitamin C and B vitamins), but WHY we can't, what affect the deficiency is having on our illness, and then, how to fix it, has been ignored thus far. This is something I feel is crucial in understanding IC and in helping our bodies heal from IC.

When it comes to stress and IC, I feel there is a huge connection between our adrenal glands, a lack of B complex vitamins and a lack of vitamin C. The adrenal glands are our stress glands. They protect us from every kind of stress to our body. These two small glands that sit on top of our kidneys are unable to distinguish between physical and psychological stress. In either case, during times of stress, our adrenals send hormones and chemicals to the organs that counteract stress. Sending out these hormones and chemicals at a faster pace during stress cannot be maintained for long periods without exhausting the supply of nutrients that feed the adrenals. Adrenal fatigue can lead to chronic fatigue and/or immune suppression, which can then lead to chronic infections, allergies, and multiple chemical sensitivities. Something I found EXTREMELY interesting is what Donald LePore, ND says in his book "The Ultimate Healing System", "In our research we have found that when adrenal glands become exhausted, the person immediately becomes allergic to citrus fruits (lemons, limes, oranges, grapefruits, tomatoes, pineapple, cantaloupe) and all the bioflavonoids."[1] When I read that, all I could think was...that's us! It is not surprising that the nutrients needed to correct this condition are B5 (Pantothenic acid) and B3 (niacin)[2], supplements that IC patients typically cannot tolerate.

Pantothenic acid, one of the B complex vitamins, stimulates the production of adrenal hormones. It is essential during any type of stress as it provides adrenal support and helps prevent adrenal exhaustion.[3] In fact, the body's requirement for Pantothenic acid increases during times of illness, stress, or exposure to toxins, all of which, in my opinion, describe the state of most IC patients. All of the B complex vitamins are necessary for the general health of the adrenals and can help guard against allergic reactions. When our adrenals are undernourished and unable to produce the hormone aldosterone, it can cause fatigue and exhaustion when the body is under stress.[4] It is so interesting to me that some IC patients have chronic fatigue and others of us seem to run on adrenaline all the time. (I was an example of the latter.) I'm not sure exactly why that is other than it has something to do with the proper functioning of our adrenal glands. Pantothenic acid is also directly related to the production of natural cortisone, which is nature's anti-inflammatory.[5] "Aching joints are one sign that the adrenals are exhausted, too exhausted to produce the hormone that prevents pain and inflammation."[7] IC patients, with their inflamed bladders also tend to have inflammation elsewhere in the body, including the joints. Some say that adrenal fatigue can be a cause and an effect of leaky gut syndrome and it makes me wonder about our leaky bladders.

IC patients are also typically deficient in vitamin C. Some people can take buffered C (sometimes called Ester C), but others can't even tolerate that. Vitamin C (ascorbic acid) is essential for the production of the adrenal hormone that protects the body against stress. In fact, the largest concentration of vitamin C in the body is in the adrenal glands.[8]

17

What is also extremely interesting is that "chemically sensitive people lose more vitamin C from the kidneys than people who have no chemical sensitivities."[9] Most IC patients are unable to take vitamin C or tolerate citrus fruits. Both typically cause burning pain in the bladder. And because many of us are chemically sensitive, we are also losing what small amounts of vitamin C we might be getting from our foods through our kidneys. (By the way, smoking cigarettes further depletes the body of vitamin C.) Then add stress to this situation and that will use up whatever tiny amounts of vitamin C (and B complex) we do have in our system in order to try and produce the hormones needed to protect our body from stress. This then further depletes the adrenal glands to where they probably can't even produce this protective hormone anymore. Also significant to IC, in my opinion, is that the adrenal glands also help maintain salt levels in the blood, maintain blood pressure, help control kidney function and control overall fluid concentrations in the body. **IC patients have a deficiency and intolerance to both major vitamins (C and B complex) that are essential to the proper functioning of the adrenal glands.**

According to a study published in the June 1999 issue of Urology, "Norepinephrine was found to be elevated in the urine from patients with IC compared with urine from normal controls. This would be consistent with increased sympathetic (adrenergic) activity, since stress is associated with symptom increase in some patients with IC."[10] It was noted that treatments such as Elmiron, DMSO, or a combination thereof, had no effect on the elevated levels in IC patients. Also interesting to note is that many IC patients have trouble with Novocain at the dentist and/or other medications that contain norepinephrine.

A body full of toxins is a major stress on the adrenal glands and the entire glandular system. It is not just the adrenals that are affected. When there is trouble with one gland, it can affect all the others. Many IC patients have thyroid problems, men with IC have prostate gland problems, and though probably not as common, there are some of us who have problems with other glands (e.g., the pituitary or pancreas).

(By the way, hypothyroidism can also exhaust the adrenals as they work overtime attempting to compensate for the malfunctioning of the thyroid.) Problems with the female sex glands (e.g., the ovaries) are another common thread among IC patients. There are many of us who have, or have had, cysts on our ovaries, fibroids, endometriosis, etc. Many IC patients have had hysterectomies. In fact, many of us experienced the onset of our IC after surgical procedures to correct the aforementioned problems.

Some alternative health practitioners believe that the body stores toxins first, in places that are not essential to sustain the life of the body. The female organs, for example, are one place where mercury is known to "collect" or be stored when the body is unable to process it all out. Some feel that opening up the body through surgery to remove the fibroids, cysts, endometriosis, scar tissue, etc., will not "cure", but only move the problem. In other words, the toxins will go elsewhere and cause other problems within the body and/or it will simply come right back. The surgery can sometimes cause a release of toxins that the body isn't prepared for and then further symptoms arise. I believe this might be the phenomenon we see at the onset of IC for some people who had these types of surgeries and also when they remove an IC bladder.

A body full of toxins also greatly affects the lymphatic system. Swollen lymph glands are indicative of either infection or an accumulation of toxins that the lymphatic system is unable to process and eliminate.[11] Many IC patients have swollen lymph glands. I had them the entire time I had IC and they were one of the last things to go down as I got better. Many of us have tender or swollen glands under our arms, at the top of our legs in the groin area, and on our neck. The lymphatic system is vital to the health of our body. It carries nutrients throughout the body and also removes waste material from all the tissues. The lymph fluid is able to go deep into tissues to pick up toxins in the form of acids and mucous which need to be eliminated. The toxins are then passed through the eliminative channels of the lymph glands and dumped into the blood stream where they are transported to the colon, kidneys, lungs or skin to be eliminated. When the lymph glands are full of toxins, the body will be filled with acids and mucous. It can promote fluid retention, loss of energy, constipation, congested sinuses, low back pain, body aches and pains, and can be the beginning of many diseases.[12]

According to a study done at the Department of Urology at Temple University School of Medicine, compared to the general population, IC patients are 100 times more likely to have inflammatory bowel disease. In fact, this same study concluded that allergies, IBS, sensitive skin, and fibromyalgia all have "an increased association with interstitial cystitis".[13] It is my opinion that all of these common symptoms/illnesses are rooted in the same toxic body. We all experience different variations of these (and other) symptoms just as we all have different levels of toxicity. One person will have a weakness where another will not.

Naturally, a toxic body puts a tremendous strain on the liver, which is a major organ of detoxification. The liver's job is to detoxify all of the synthetic chemicals we eat, the pharmaceutical medications we take, the heavy metals we are exposed to, etc., and even the toxins that are produced within the body. When the liver is overburdened in trying to expel poisons it puts an overload on the kidneys. There are some people who theorize that IC is caused by a toxic substance coming from the kidneys.

Among many other things, the liver regulates the balance of sex hormones, thyroid hormones, cortisone and other adrenal hormones. It does this by inactivating and eliminating hormones through the bile or urine. If the liver fails to remove them efficiently, it can cause an accumulation in the tissues that can lead to abnormal growths such as fibroids, ovarian cysts, endometriosis, breast cysts and tumors, prostate enlargement and prostate cancer. Many people believe that "estrogen dominance" (or lack of progesterone to balance the estrogen) is the cause of many female problems including bloating, PMS, breast tenderness, cysts, fibroids, etc. If the liver is congested with toxins and is unable to balance the hormones effectively, it can cause many problems throughout the body. Again, where some people will have an imbalance in one direction, others might have an imbalance in the other.

If the liver is congested with fats or accumulated toxins, it cannot produce the enzyme histaminase, which is the body's protection against allergies. And again, the two major vitamins that IC patients often have trouble with, B complex and vitamin C, are both essential for the liver to detoxify. If the liver is not producing enough bile because it is congested with toxins, digestion will be difficult and a toxic colon can result.

A toxic body (and toxic colon) does not absorb nutrition.

Most IC patients have a toxic colon, often with yeast overgrowth, but certainly not always. Irritable Bowel Syndrome is VERY common among IC patients. So common in fact, that with the exception of those with very mild IC, I don't think I even know an IC patient that doesn't have at least some symptoms of an irritable bowel (even if they haven't been formally diagnosed with IBS). Many IC patients feel that their IBS symptoms are related to their IC symptoms. For example, when their IBS is "flared", so is their IC. Or following a bowel movement, there is a burning sensation experienced in the bladder and urethra. Or when constipated, their IC symptoms are much worse. Or when under stress, both their IBS and IC will get worse. A toxic colon is closely linked to sinus congestion and also to allergies, both of which are found readily among IC patients. Symptoms such as frequent diarrhea and/or constipation, gas, bloating, and cramping are all signs of a toxic colon.

Intestinal toxicity is intimately related to immune dysfunction. The small and large intestine are actually part of the immune system. It is the mucous layers of the intestines that trap toxins and pathogens and act as a first line of defense against infection and disease. If our body is unable to remove toxins through normal excretion, which is the body's

21

first line of defense, it will take additional steps to protect itself. This is where the "itises" come in (e.g., colitis, sinusitis, gastritis, bronchitis, cystitis). "Itis" stands for inflammation. Inflammation is a part of our body's healing defense. It's the body's most intense effort to cleanse and restore itself. With inflammation, the toxins in the body have usually been concentrated in a particular organ or area of the body for a massive elimination effort. The area becomes inflamed due to the constant irritation from toxic material and then we are usually diagnosed with one of the "itises". In our case, interstitial cystitis, inflammation of the bladder wall. Many of us also have more widespread inflammation such as with fibromyalgia or lupus, or else we have several separate locations where we have inflammation such as the gums, the vulva area (Vulvodynia), the intestines, and/or the sinuses.

Do I still think that bacteria are (or can be) involved in IC or that systemic candida is (or can be) involved? Yes I do and here is why. **The toxic body of an IC patient provides the perfect environment for bacteria and fungus to thrive.** Bacteria are present in, on, and around the body all the time. It's when the body is weakened that it will become vulnerable to infection. The more toxic the body, the more likely that the IC patient will have bacteria, fungus, viruses, etc. involved in their IC. The more toxic the body, the weaker will be the immune system. The more toxic the body, the more IC-related symptoms arise.

What else does the toxic body promote? In other words, if the body is toxic what symptoms typically occur? A huge variety of seemingly unrelated symptoms can occur. And though it will be different for everyone, there are some similar symptoms of people with a toxic body.

The following is a list of symptoms common for a toxic body.
Allergies of all kinds
Sensitive to environment (especially things like chemicals, perfume, synthetics, paint and exhaust fumes)

Mucous membrane problems
Muscle aches and joint pain
Digestive problems
Bloating
Back pain (especially lower back pain due to a toxic colon and constipation)
Sore throat and nasal congestion (often linked to a toxic colon and/or allergies)
Immune system weakness
Depression and/or anxiety
Constipation and/or diarrhea
Insomnia
Tight or stiff neck
Headaches
Fatigue
Bad breathe and coated tongue
Itching with no rash
Skin problems (e.g., acne, hives, mysterious rashes, etc.)

Granted, the above symptoms can have a multitude of causes, but nevertheless they are often present when the body is toxic. And interestingly enough, many of these symptoms coincide with the most common IC and IC-related symptoms. The mucous membranes are a good example. Healthy mucous membranes protect our organs from invasion by bacteria. Allergies and colds, for example, are the body's way of eliminating toxins by way of the mucous membranes. It is actually nature's way of protecting and cleansing the body of unwanted irritants (allergens, bacteria, or toxins). But when the body is overloaded with toxins and is unable to eliminate them all through the natural eliminative organs (e.g., the kidneys, colon, lungs, and skin), stress is then added to the mucous membranes. Healthy mucous membranes prevent undigested proteins and toxins from entering the bloodstream and causing allergies.[14] With IC, we don't have healthy mucous membranes (the bladder lining, the intestines, the mouth, the sinuses, the vaginal area, etc.) and I don't believe we have healthy adrenal function either. It is interesting to note that the job of the adrenal glands is to provide hormones that render foreign protein harmless.[15] The reason I find it so interesting is because of some of the current IC research results. For example, Dr. Susan Keay's research suggests that there is a protein in the urine of IC patients that they call the "antiproliferative factor" or APF that is not present in the urine of controls (i.e., non-IC patients). They believe this protein inhibits the normal growth of cells that line the bladder surface. In other words, because this protein is present in the urine, our bladders cannot repair themselves normally.[16] Also, Dr. S. Grant Mulholland of Philadelphia has identified a glycoprotein called GP51 that he feels might play a role in bladder permeability in IC patients. There are lower levels of this protein in IC patients compared to controls. It is hypothesized that if the GP51 levels could be increased that it would decrease bladder symptoms.[17] Anyway, I just thought that was interesting.

Another good example is allergies and sensitivities.

A toxic body promotes allergies and sensitivities.

This is the reason, I believe, why most of us become chemically sensitive and/or develop allergies. It is my opinion that our bodies simply cannot take any more additional chemicals/poisons/toxins. Whether they come from food, the environment, or medications, it doesn't matter. We are very SENSITIVE. Sensitive to medications and supplements, sensitive to cold and heat, sensitive to smells, sensitive to everything. I think this is VERY important to recognize when treating IC.

I believe that many of our differences in symptoms and in how we react to different treatments is based in part on the fact that we all develop different allergies/sensitivities. These different allergies are a major reason why we are all different in terms of what foods, medications, vitamins, and herbs that we can tolerate. Different treatments work for different people depending, in part, on their particular allergies/sensitivities. The same medication that helps one IC patient might put another one in the hospital with an allergic reaction. Sometimes we can take a medication or herb for a while and it helps us, and then all of a sudden it stops helping us and/or we become allergic to it. We can develop allergies almost instantaneously and seemingly spontaneously, so we have to be very careful. Many times, actually more often than not, the IC patient will not be aware of ALL of their allergies/sensitivities. This might be a good time to point out that neither is their doctor. I think this is VERY important to recognize when treating IC.

Because I see the IC patient as having a toxic body with irritated and inflamed tissues in the bladder and elsewhere, I have to admit that I don't believe invasive treatments are the answer. I recognize that there are some IC patients who have found relief in bladder instillations and distensions (albeit temporary); they still in fact do provide relief for some people. Personally, I would never deny an IC patient any option for relief of any kind no matter how temporary. But from my perspective they are simply not the approach I would take. Not only do I come from the perspective that God did not intend us to stick things into our bladders, I believe that doing so when the bladder is already inflamed, sore, irritated, bleeding, etc. is not a good thing; it is not a healing thing to do in my opinion. I realize that if you instill a numbing medication or anti-inflammatory medication that it will squelch symptoms for a time. And therefore, some can argue that they have their place in IC treatments. But from my perspective, invasive procedures offer more risk. More risk for infection and more risk of further irritation to an already inflamed and irritated bladder (and urethra). I know many IC patients who have gotten worse because of the invasive treatments that were done to them. Some feel damaged beyond repair, that their bladders will never be the same. I know that most people were never told that there was even a risk that they could get worse from these treatments. Again, this is where talking to other IC patients can be extremely helpful. IC patients will truthfully share their opinions because they have nothing to gain or lose by doing so.

25

I also believe a latex allergy is something else that IC patients need to be concerned about if they decide to go the route of bladder instillations. Latex allergies can be a very serious thing and most people don't know if they are allergic to latex or not. If you can find out before using catheters, latex gloves, condoms, etc., you will be doing yourself a huge favor. Due to IC patients' extreme sensitivity and our tendency to develop allergies, I believe a latex allergy is something that we should be checked for prior to these types of treatments and procedures that use catheters. This is also important because one of the fairly common ways that people get IC is after exposure to catheters. Some people believe this is due to infection being introduced via the catheter, but it could also be due to an allergic reaction to latex. I think all of these things are VERY important to recognize when treating IC.

On top of all the toxins that we are exposed to on a daily basis, it is considered normal in our society that when we get sick, we take a pill. We ingest synthetic, chemical medications that we expect to "make us better". Pharmaceutical medications can no doubt be fantastic for crisis situations. They often work quickly to cover symptoms and/or provide relief of some kind, and I know that we are all very grateful for them. But for long-term health care, for chronic illness, these chemical medications can often cause more problems. These medications are often known to cause side effects. We are usually (hopefully) informed of these side effects by our doctor or when we pick up our prescriptions. We think of this as "to be expected". We think of this as normal. The side effects of medications are often a risk that we are fully willing to take because they come "doctor recommended" and are "FDA approved". Sometimes a dependence of the body on the chemical medication can occur. Sometimes the situation can become worse than it was before the pill was ever taken. Very often a mixture of medications has the person confused with no idea of what is working and what isn't. I think, with IC, this is often the case. It is not uncommon for an IC patient to be taking some combination of the following medications...pain medications, anti-depressants, muscle relaxants, anti-histamines, antibiotics, anti-inflammatories, analgesics, and possibly additional medications for other conditions. Because I see the IC patient as having a toxic body, I believe then that synthetic, chemical medications are further adding to that toxicity and often making the situation worse. It may appear that they are helping because they are helping to cover or mask symptoms, but in reality they might be making the situation worse. In my opinion, this can often be the case with IC. Adding chemicals to an already toxic body will not cure IC. This is not a guess. It has been proven by medical science that has been unable to "cure" IC thus far. Remissions can occur for some people, yes. Often, in my opinion, in spite of the medications and/or invasive procedures and sometimes due to a temporary covering of symptoms. But is it still remission when "flares" still occur? When a special diet still must be adhered to? When things are better than they were, but not "normal"? Or is remission a return to health? I am not writing this to criticize, but rather to point out that maybe, just possibly, the medical approach to IC is not helping and is possibly even hurting some IC patients. It is just something I hope that doctors might consider someday and something that I hope you might consider right now.

Don't get me wrong. If you have had great success with the medical approach to healing IC, then I think that's wonderful. Whatever works for you, I think is great. I am just talking to those people who haven't had such great success with the medical approach and/or who would like to try a more natural approach to healing their IC. I have a feeling that those will be the people most likely to be reading this book.

Something else I feel is important to recognize when treating IC is that, in my opinion, IC patients are not absorbing nutrition. Not only are we eating under a restricted diet, but also the nutrition or food that we *are* getting is not necessarily being absorbed. Being toxic and not absorbing the vitamins and minerals we need also accounts, in my opinion, for many of the "extra" symptoms that can come with IC such as MVP (a lack of potassium can result in abnormal heart rhythms), difficulty with anxiety (a lack of B vitamins), bloating (a lack of B6 and/or potassium), anemia (a lack of iron), etc. Instead of medicating the symptom, I think it would be more helpful to determine whether a vitamin or mineral deficiency might be causing the problem. I will even go so far as to suggest that this might very often be the case. Adding synthetic medications will only cover the symptoms and cause more problems. They will be putting even more strain on already strained organs such as the kidneys and liver for example, which are absolutely crucial in our body's ability to filter toxins and waste. (I don't find it coincidental that IC patients who take Elmiron are asked to have their liver and kidneys tested every 3-6 months.) If an IC patient is experiencing an irregular heartbeat and is told that they have MVP, they will then be told to take antibiotics every time they go to the dentist. They are taking the antibiotics for "preventative" measures, but doing so without having an infection present, is killing even more beneficial bacteria in the colon and throwing off the balance of intestinal flora even further. (Naturally I am not suggesting that someone with MVP not take antibiotics prior to going to the dentist. Though I would suggest including acidophilus to counteract the negative effects of the antibiotics.) If an IC patient is having trouble with anxiety, a medical doctor doesn't usually consider that it's due to a lack of B complex vitamins so he/she prescribes an anti-anxiety medication. Or if an IC patient experiences depression (which can also be a symptom of a toxic body), the person will most likely be given Prozac or some such anti-depressant. Covering up symptoms of a toxic body with medications and covering up symptoms that are occurring due to a lack of vitamins/minerals, to me, is not going to help matters. Instead we are becoming even more toxic and therefore even less able to absorb the nutrition that we so desperately need. Our body becomes even more taxed and overworked trying to cleanse itself of all the additional toxins that the medications are providing. It is my belief that our symptoms begin because the body is unable to process out all the toxic waste to begin with and then when it reacts with symptoms, we end up medicating ourselves even more and thus making the situation even worse. I think this is VERY important to recognize when treating IC.

I believe that an IC patient's body is out of balance in many ways. The intestinal flora is very often (nearly always) out of balance. There is usually a problem with the acid/alkaline balance in the body. Often the hormones, blood sugar, and blood pressure are also out of balance. Another thing that I have found is that the potassium/sodium balance is very often out of whack in an IC patients' body. Many IC patients cannot tolerate foods that contain potassium or are told to avoid potassium rich foods and are therefore not getting enough potassium into their body. Plus there are many who take some form of laxative or are experiencing diarrhea fairly often and are loosing potassium this way as well. This imbalance can show itself in the form of swelling and I believe it is one major component of the IC-related edema for some people. Unfortunately what is happening is that many doctors are then giving the IC patients diuretics, which in my opinion are further promoting the problem because diuretics further deplete the body of potassium. It is my opinion that all of these various imbalances are being caused by the toxicity within the body affecting different organs and body systems. Again, it will be different for different people. But in many ways, getting well and staying well, is about getting the body back into balance.

The level of toxicity in each IC patient varies and therefore so will the "course" of their illness. I believe this is the reason why some IC patients seem to level off in terms of their symptoms for years maybe and then all of a sudden something might happen (major stress, another illness, an infection of some kind, a change in their environment even) and their IC will get much worse. It's why some IC patients feel that IC is a progressive disease because theirs got progressively worse over time. And then some people feel strongly that IC is *not* progressive because they were worse symptom-wise when they first got diagnosed, but maybe are doing about the same or better since then. And then there are those IC patients who seem to go into spontaneous remissions having no idea why their IC symptoms disappeared. Thrilled as they are, they're not sure what happened. Something mysteriously put them back into balance. I feel these various scenarios are in great part due to the level of toxicity in the body of the IC patient. How much is their body able to efficiently eliminate and how much more toxicity is being added? How much nutrition are they getting into their body and how much are they absorbing? How many different medications are they adding to their body that their body then has to process out? How many more stressors are being added to their body and/or their life? All of these things, in my opinion, will influence the "course" of their illness.

The various symptoms among us are not only dependent upon our different allergies/sensitivities, but also on our individual body weaknesses and the level of toxicity throughout our bodies. As I said earlier, I believe that although IC manifests itself in different ways for each individual, we do have the toxic body in common. And in my opinion, from that starting point, we can develop a healing plan; a SAFE healing plan that can be tailored to each individual. A healing plan that gets to the root of the problem instead of one that covers up symptoms; one that will return an individual to normal health. A healing plan for IC patients, in my opinion should take into consideration our multiple (most likely unknown to the individual) allergies/sensitivities. It should take into consideration that we are full of poison and very toxic, and therefore very (sometimes EXTREMELY) sensitive. It should take into consideration that some IC patients DO in fact have bacteria, fungus and viruses involved in their IC (whether IC on the whole is caused by bacteria or not). It should take into account that IC is not just a bladder disease. It is my opinion that IC treatments should "first do no harm". And it is also my opinion that we should "revere the laws of nature" and the natural healing ability of our own bodies.

Steps Along the Path

There is so very much hope for you to get well regardless of how severe your IC is in this moment and regardless of how long you have suffered with this disease. I'm telling you, there is still hope. There are many ways to return to a state of health whether you have a mild, moderate, or severe case of IC. And please, I don't want you to just believe me on any of this. Talk to other IC patients. Read about the toxic body from other sources and decide for yourself if this is you; if this feels like your situation. Decide for yourself if this perspective of IC feels right to you. I feel strongly that this is the approach to take in order to get well, but naturally I am a bit biased because this is the approach that worked for me. So I want you to keep that in mind too. But when you start looking at IC based on the perspective of the toxic body, I'm telling you, a lot of the mystery and differences among us start to make a lot more sense. I really believe that the toxic body is what makes IC so confusing; it's why we're all different, it's why IC is not just one thing, and it's why IC can be everything. Our toxicity is also what causes us to be so sensitive and allergy prone, thus creating even more differences between us.

After reading *To Wake In Tears*, people have been writing and calling me asking..."Now what should I do? What would you do if you were in my shoes? What should I do first? How do I go about this? I know we're all different, I know you're not a doctor, but HELP!" Trying to heal from IC can be so overwhelming. Especially if you want to take a more natural approach because there are so many options. There are so many choices and it's difficult to know who to listen to. Often we have so many things physically wrong with us at the same time, we barely know where to start. And at the same time, most of us probably know very little about herbs and alternative treatments and are therefore starting from ground zero in terms of knowing what to do. I have tried to somehow simplify the process of what I did, the steps I took to get well. I hope they might be able to serve as a guideline to help you come up with a healing plan of your own based on your individual situation and of course based on what you feel most comfortable with.

I feel the need to preface the following with so many things. For example, there is nobody more qualified to determine what you should do for your IC than you are. Neither myself, nor anyone else can know your body, your symptoms and what is possibly affecting you, the way you can. And only you can determine what your perspective of IC is; what you believe is causing *your* IC. The following is based on my perspective. It is a holistic, natural approach that does not require invasive procedures or unnecessary pain. I often wonder why pain is not more of a consideration in traditional medicine's approach to IC. From the older chlorpactin instillations and urethral dilations to the newer potassium sensitivity test or cayenne pepper treatment, I don't understand why so many IC treatments and diagnostic procedures have to involve additional pain. I was in so much pain with my IC that I could not fathom doing these treatments. I give a lot of credit to those of you who have given them a shot. As scary as it is to attempt to heal yourself naturally and investigate alternative treatments for IC, I have to be honest and say that I was much more afraid to try the medical treatments. Again, we all have to do what we feel most comfortable with.

The following are seven major steps to recovering from Interstitial Cystitis. These are steps I took myself and steps I've watched others take to recover as well. I strongly believe that our bodies have the ability to heal themselves if given the chance. I also strongly believe that we must do everything we can to support the body's healing, as well as remove any and all obstacles possible so that our body has a chance to heal itself. As I said earlier, I don't believe invasive treatments are the way to go with IC. I also don't believe that adding synthetic chemicals to an already overly toxic body is going to promote healing. And I don't believe treating the bladder and ignoring the rest of the body will return you to a state of normal health. I do believe that there are certain important steps you can take to help soothe and cleanse your body that will actually help you to heal. I also believe it is just as important, if not more so, to remove the sources of toxins which have gotten you to this point in the first place. I also believe it's important, once you get yourself to the place where you can tolerate it, to replenish the body with nutrients. These things will give your bladder and body the chance to heal itself. You might want to read through all the steps first because some of them you may need to do in a different order or even simultaneously.

Step 1 - Get out of pain

Before anything else, we need to get ourselves out of pain. This is most important. We can't think straight when we're in pain or when we're so incredibly uncomfortable with all the other symptoms of IC. Before making any treatment decisions, it is very important to be out of pain so that you can think clearly and make a wise choice. My friend Barb Willis taught me this. She has suffered from IC and all of it's horrendous other symptoms for over 25 years and she reminds us how she had made some bad treatment choices years ago just out of desperation. Because she was in so much pain she was willing to let the doctors, or whoever, do just about anything to her. She was in pain while at the doctor's office, saying okay to whatever they said they wanted to do to her. How many of us have done that? If she hadn't been feeling so desperate because of the pain, she could have taken time to research the treatment further, examine all of her options, and then decide what to do. Barb learned her lesson the hard way and hopes that you won't have to make the same mistake. Get out of pain before you decide to do anything at all, treatment-wise, for your IC.

A lot of IC patients have trouble getting pain medication from their urologist. I'm not sure exactly why urologists don't treat the pain of IC, but I do know that many of them don't. I don't know if it's because they don't understand how painful it is or because they are afraid they will get in trouble prescribing pain medications. Whatever the reason, please know that you're not alone if you've had trouble getting something to take for pain. Thankfully, there are doctors who are trained to treat pain and are even more aware of different types of pain medications than a regular doctor might be. If your urologist won't treat your pain (which unfortunately most don't or won't), it's very important to find a doctor who will. Whether you go to an internist or a pain doctor, find someone right away who will understand how incredibly painful IC can be. For those with severe IC, the pain is very comparable to end stage cancer pain. Even someone with a moderate case of IC can have unbelievable pain. Find someone who understands that the pain is not in your head and get yourself out of pain as soon as possible. We don't deserve to suffer just because certain doctors are unwilling to recognize that IC pain is real or just because it doesn't fall under the category heading of things that they are willing to treat.

Pain is another form of physical stress to the body. Our bodies can't even begin to heal while they are suffering in pain. Throughout your healing you will need to keep yourself out of pain as much as possible. There are natural ways to deal with pain, but initially, most likely you will need to take some type of prescription medication. As you begin to heal your bladder and the rest of your body, your need for the synthetic medications will decrease until you won't have to take them anymore. One thing that will help very much in this area is the next step.

Step 2 - Soothe your insides

Soothe your insides, especially your bladder. This is something you will find helpful right away and this is also a "step" you will need to do all throughout your healing. There are so many different things you can use to help soothe your insides. In Sections 4 and 5 of this book you will find many herbs and natural products that can help in this area. But for now I just want to stress the importance of soothing. Most likely you are in the situation right now where your bladder lining, urethra, and/or the entire vaginal area (or prostate area for the guys) is inflamed and irritated. Possibly your intestines are a mess and your stomach as well. You might even have a situation where your tongue is burning and your throat hurts all the time. It is my personal opinion that giving your bladder and body soothing things is one of the smartest things you can do throughout the entire time you're healing from IC. I believe our body, through our symptoms, is actually crying out to be soothed. That's what all the pain, inflammation, and irritation are telling us. Just as very dry, raw, sunburned or inflamed skin cries out to be soothed with aloe vera or cocoa butter or whatever, so is your bladder crying out to be soothed with something. Anything! I mean, if a body could scream at the top of it's lungs in words that we could understand, our bodies would be screaming SOOTHE ME, SOOTHE ME!! Because we are all different, you will need to experiment a little to find which ones will help you, but at least there are several different options to choose from. Take your pick of various herbs and natural products that have a demulcent quality, as well as those that de-acidify your system. (see sections 4 & 5) And if you're in an emergency situation right now, have your doctor write you a prescription for Pyridium or something to help you get through the immediate crisis. Even if you choose to go a more natural route to healing, it doesn't mean that certain medications short term can't provide you some relief. Some people, thinking I would only do "alternative" natural stuff, have asked me if I think it's bad to take pain medications or something like Pyridium, etc. and the answer is no. I think medications can serve a purpose in the short term that can be extremely helpful. I just don't think they are a good long-term solution is all. As I've said before, I am not against ANY form of IC treatment that brings a person relief. Anybody who has IC I'm sure feels the same way.

Step 3 - Determine your present situation

You will need to be able to decide whether you are strong enough physically, and whether your bladder is well enough, to handle some of the next steps. You are the only one who will really know that. No one can tell you what you can tolerate. No doctor, no acupuncturist, no herbologist, no urologist; no one but you. No one can FEEL you like you can. Each time you take a medication or herb, or even eat something, only YOU can be the one to decide whether it is hurting you or not.

You will have to feel your way through your healing.

You will have to not only pay attention to how you feel, but to trust those feelings. And you will not only have to trust your feelings, but also act on them. For example, many IC patients, after trying a new herb or medication, feel like they might be getting worse from it. So they call the doctor or alternative healthcare provider and are told that it "couldn't be the herb or medication" or that they should "continue on with the protocol". So they continue taking the herb or medication. Instead of listening to their own inner knowing, their own physical feelings, they will take the word of someone else instead. I'll say it again, please trust yourself and your physical symptoms over what anyone else is telling you to do, including me. Only you can protect yourself from additional harm.

Keeping track of what you are doing and how you are feeling will help you a lot. It will help you know whether what you are doing is helping or hurting, whether you are improving or going backwards, whether you are on the right path. Writing it down and keeping track will allow you to be able to see the patterns of your symptoms as you ovulate or go through your menstrual cycle, for example, or as you are under additional stress or eating something new. You will be able to make wiser choices. You will have to be the one to determine where you are with your IC, now and throughout your healing. Again, only you will be able to discover how much your bladder and body can tolerate. Please keep that in mind when choosing from the various options available.

You are probably going to want to deal with your most severe symptoms first. You will need to look to your own body to determine which organs are most affected right now and what is the priority for you to deal with. Everyone will be different. It might be your bladder (for many of you it will be) or it might be your fibro symptoms (muscle and joint pain). It could be both. Or maybe right now your glands are hugely swollen and you have an infection in your mouth and an earache, but your bladder is calm for the moment. You get the idea. With IC, we have to "go with the flow" and deal with our symptoms as they come up because God knows new ones seem to come up all the time. At this point I would make a list of the main organs you're having trouble with (for example, kidneys, bladder, thyroid, liver, and lungs or bladder, lymph glands, intestines and stomach). I'm sure you get the idea. A list of all the symptoms you have right now is also a good idea and will lead you to the list of organs that are affected. Having this list will help you begin to develop your healing plan. In the next sections you will be able to choose from many herbs, natural products, and alternative treatments to help soothe and support these various organs.

Determine what "stage" of IC you're in right now. (By the way, these are just "stages" that I've noticed among IC patients. They are not "medical" stages.) For example, is your body and bladder all torn down right now? If you're losing a lot of weight no matter what you eat or because you can barely eat, yet you have a big bloated belly and can barely stand up straight from the pain because your bladder is a mess right now, then I would consider you in a "torn down" stage. (Initially, this was me.) Maybe you're bleeding right now from either the bladder or the intestines or both. If this is your situation, I would consider that your organs are beat up and exhausted. It is my opinion that you need to be doing a lot of soothing and gentle nourishment before you can go further. In other words, you wouldn't want to jump right into cleansing (step 6) because your body and bladder probably couldn't tolerate that right now. If you're bloated all over your body (edema) and/or your fibromyalgia symptoms are acting up, but you have your bladder symptoms somewhat under control at the moment, I'd consider you at a different stage of IC that, to be honest, I have no particular name for. (By the way, later on, this was me.) If you are at this stage, then you might want to consider some gentle cleansing (and also some soothing things to do while you're cleansing). Maybe you are functioning in life right now (able to work and do some form of exercise for example) but you still have bladder symptoms, bloating in the pelvic area, and maybe a couple of other non-debilitating-type symptoms and you are just maintaining right now. Or maybe you have horrible bladder symptoms but don't notice that you have any other symptoms right now. I am just saying these examples in general right now so that you see how we are not all at the same point in our IC. You are going to want to devise your healing plan based upon where you are in the moment. Not on what is right for other people, but what is right for you.

In determining your situation, I would also make a list of the medications you are taking. To the extent that you can, I would recommend finding out what these various medications are doing to your body. In other words, are they working with each other or against each other? Are you experiencing symptoms ("side effects") being caused by the combination of medications you are on or even from one of the medications? Or are the symptoms you are experiencing "your own"? In other words, are you able to distinguish between your "natural" symptoms due to IC and the symptoms/side effects being caused by the medications? Are the medications you are taking depleting your body of certain vitamins and minerals? All I'm saying here is maybe you know the answers to these questions and maybe you don't. When I was taking medications for my IC, I didn't have a clue. I didn't know much about the medications and I certainly had no idea what they were doing to my body. I just prayed that when I took them I wouldn't experience any of the side effects listed on the printout

I got from the pharmacy. And then I would pray that it would work and that I'd at least find some relief by taking them. I am not telling you to stop taking your medicine that the doctor gave you. What I'm saying is to find out what the medications you are taking are doing to your body. I would also consider that the medications are adding more toxins/chemicals to your body that your body then has to filter out through the kidneys and liver, for example, and ultimately through the intestines and bladder. No matter how helpful these medications are at covering symptoms, they are also putting more stress and strain on the body because after we take them, we then have to process them out. It is my opinion that with IC, where all the eliminative organs are, or can be, affected, that we should pay attention to this fact. And if the medications cause constipation, for example, you might consider that they are causing you to "hold in" even more toxins and waste. Aside from the extra pressure on the bladder, I think this "holding in of the toxins" is why many of us feel even worse when constipated. Even if you don't think the root cause of IC has anything to do with a toxic body and you totally disagree with my perspective, it would still be wise (in my opinion) to at least find out what these synthetic chemicals are doing to your body. You will have to be the one to decide if you want to be on the medication indefinitely. In other words, are you comfortable being on these medications long term? I have a feeling most people reading this are thinking NO WAY do I want to take this stuff the rest of my life. But at the same time, you're probably thinking, what choice do I have? (That's what I thought anyway.) Well right now, maybe you don't have a choice. But from my perspective, if you don't right now, you WILL or CAN have a choice later on down the line. For one thing, there are often natural alternatives to synthetic pharmaceutical medications. And for another, if you get to the root of the problem and your body heals, you won't need the medications any more.

Determine your present situation in terms of whether you have an infection, bacterial, fungal, or viral, going on right now. You might be reading this feeling like you have an infection that never quite went away. Maybe you have had repeated infections and the last one just never went away, so you were put on various antibiotics, and still you

39

don't feel right. Now you have been told that you have IC and that you don't have an infection. But you still feel infected. Maybe you have other symptoms of infection, like swollen glands, a low-grade fever, and chills. Maybe you have read through all the IC literature and read both sides of the bacteria debate and you still feel strongly like your IC is caused by infection. I know this was how I felt. I didn't have repeated bladder infections but I did have one huge bladder/kidney infection following surgery and it never seemed to go away. I still felt like I was infected and that I had all the symptoms of infection, even though the normal 2-3 day culture at the doctor's office didn't show infection. I still felt like it was the cause of my IC at the time. If this is how you feel in your present situation, you might consider having your urine cultured by Dr. Paul Fugazzotto at the Cystitis Research Center, for example, to find out if he finds bacteria in your sample. He cultures the urine with a more sophisticated broth culture that he grows for 5-7 days. His perspective is that just because the bacteria doesn't grow in the allotted 2-3 day time slot that our labs generally allow, doesn't mean that the bacteria is not there. To reach Dr. Fugazzotto you can call 1-605-342-8989 or write to the Cystitis Research Center at 4021 Wonderland Dr., Rapid City, South Dakota 57702.

Even if you don't believe bacteria causes IC, you probably know that having IC makes one more prone to getting bladder infections because our bladders are compromised. Not only bladder infections, but with a compromised immune system we are more prone to infections of all kinds. And so there are times where you might need to decide whether or not you have an infection going on. So how do you do that? As you know, most of the time with IC it is VERY tough to tell if you have a "regular" bladder infection or not. Some people buy those at-home UTI test kits from their pharmacy so they can check at home for infection. I could never find those so I had to go to the doctor each time to have a culture done. It can get frustrating because a lot of times nothing will show up, but then there will be times it does. I always felt stupid when nothing showed up and like they thought I was nuts coming in so often to check, but then there were the times that a huge infection would show up and I was glad I went. You can look at your symptoms to try and help you determine if you have infection going on. For example, do you have swollen glands? Do you get low-grade fevers and chills? Sounds funny, but do you "feel" infected? If you don't and/or if you've tried antibiotics in the past for your IC and they didn't help OR if you think your IC began after antibiotic use, then this is probably not the way to go for you (obviously). Some people (in my opinion) have toxicity and inflammation in their body, but they don't currently have bacterial infection present. Other people are so toxic and sick that infections keep coming back constantly. That's the situation I was in when I was first sick. I was so full of poison/toxins with my immune system severely compromised, that I was very susceptible to infection. Along with getting repeated bladder infections (which I never got prior to IC), I was catching every little thing that went around.

It will be up to you to decide if you have bacteria involved in your IC. Some people feel their IC actually started from taking antibiotics and that could very well be the case. Not only because they might possibly have systemic candida (yeast) from taking so many antibiotics (and systemic candida can mimic IC symptoms), but also some people actually had their IC symptoms start after an allergic reaction to antibiotics. This is not unheard of. I know several IC patients who have had bad reactions to Macrodantin, for example, or Bactrim. I know I had a bad reaction to sulfa antibiotics. It happened after I got IC, but I didn't know that I had IC at the time. I was still undiagnosed at that point and my doctor wanted to cover all the bases with this sulfa antibiotic because he could see that all my symptoms were pointing to infection. I believe this was the very beginning of my fibromyalgia symptoms actually. It was the first time I ever had horrible muscle and joint pain in my life.

Do I think antibiotics are the way to go in treating IC? Not necessarily and certainly not for everyone. I do think that antibiotics are helpful in certain situations for some people. Antibiotics helped me tremendously when my IC was very severe. They stopped my bladder from bleeding huge blood clots and definitely took me to a different level in terms of getting better. I will forever be indebted to Dr. Paul Fugazzotto for his help and broth culture technique. However, taking long-term antibiotics (I took them for 4 months) also caused me to develop a more serious situation with candida (yeast) and I knew I couldn't stay on antibiotics forever. I ended up looking for a more natural approach to treating systemic candida, knowing also that I couldn't take Diflucan (a prescription anti-fungal) forever either. This was really the beginning of my turning to alternative treatments for IC. Would I take antibiotics again? Yes. If I were in that same situation with my bladder bleeding and my symptoms so severe, yes, I would try them again. I had all the symptoms of infection and simply because the regular urine cultures weren't showing infection, didn't mean I didn't have infection going on. That's how I felt about it. Dr. Fugazzotto grew the culture for 7 days instead of 2-3 and he found bacteria. I felt at that time, and I think I would again, that it was the right thing for me to do. If I had to do it all over again I probably wouldn't have stayed on them for 4 months though. I would have switched to natural antibiotics sooner. And I would have taken a lot of acidophilus while I was taking the antibiotics, but I didn't know any better at the time. I probably would have done something to boost my immune system while I was taking them too, but again, I didn't know any better at the time. I didn't know that antibiotics are hard on the immune system or that the yeast situation could get that out of control. But for me, at that time, antibiotics were appropriate. At that time, for me, bacteria were involved in my symptoms, so they did help me. This will not be the case for everyone though.

It will also be up to you to determine whether or not you have systemic candida. I included a candida quiz in the Appendix to help you decide whether it might be an issue for you and whether you might need to look into it further. There are some great books out there on the subject and/or you can search the Internet and read about it there. The more you read about it, the more you will be able to determine whether candida is a factor for you. If you have mild IC symptoms or if you have taken repeated antibiotics, for example, I would look into systemic candida for a possible answer. Candida can mimic IC symptoms because candida releases toxins into the body. It is possible to be tested for systemic yeast, but you will probably have to go to an alternative type doctor to do so.

Some people believe that a virus causes IC. I'm pretty sure that is Chinese medicine's view of IC as well. And even if you don't think a virus causes IC, you may have other viruses going on while you have IC. From the flu and colds to Epstein-Barr and Herpes, many will experience a virus along with their IC. You might be among those of us who have experienced that strange phenomenon where we get the flu and our IC symptoms seem to subside, until the flu gets better and then our IC symptoms come right back. There are some IC patients who experience what they call flares and remissions. Some might attribute that to a viral component as viruses can lay dormant in the body and then flare during times of stress or a lowered immune system.

In all of the situations of infection, whether bacterial, viral, or fungal, you will have to determine whether you want to take natural or pharmaceutical medications to combat it. It is my belief that it is wise to boost the immune system regardless, no matter which route you choose. One reason is because synthetic antibiotics can wreak havoc on the immune system. Anti-fungal and the new anti-viral medications I'm sure do the same. Not only does your immune system need further support when on these "anti" medications, I would say that our immune system needs help fighting the infections to begin with. I feel that boosting the immune system so that our body can fight the infection on it's own is also wise. If you would like to fight the infection naturally, you will be able to find several natural antibiotic/antifungal herbs and natural products in sections 4 and 5.

On the other hand, what if you believe that your IC is an autoimmune disease? Then there is the issue of whether you think boosting your immune system is a good thing or not. There are two schools of thought on this. Some people believe that with autoimmune diseases, boosting the immune system is a bad thing to do. They believe this because by definition autoimmune disease is where the immune system turns on the body and starts destroying itself. It is an abnormal reaction of the body to its own tissues. But there are others who believe that one of the causes of autoimmune disease is a weakened immune system and it is therefore "confused" and needs to be strengthened in order for it to heal and begin working normally again. Many people believe that autoimmune disease is caused by either physical or emotional stress, undetected infections (bacterial, viral, parasitic, etc.), a toxic body, even vaccinations and pregnancy have been blamed. If you believe your IC is autoimmune in nature, my best advice would be to read both sides of this argument in terms of boosting the immune system and do what feels most comfortable to you.

You will have to be the one to decide whether you even believe your body is toxic or not. So how do you know if you are toxic? How can you determine whether this is true of your IC as it was for mine? And is there a way you can find out for sure? Are there tests you can have done to find out? YES! There are blood tests, hair analysis, and various other ways "alternative" doctors can test you to find out if you have a toxic body. Don't just believe me on this, check it out for yourself. You can be tested for mercury, lead, and other heavy metals. You can also be tested for candida, which we know produces toxins. You can also examine your symptoms and your situation yourself. There are signs to look for. Do you have a coated tongue (yellow, white, or even greenish coating), bad breath, and/or digestive problems? Do you smoke or take synthetic medications? Do you have metal in your mouth? Do you crave sugar and carbohydrates? Do you have food allergies and/or environmental allergies? Do you get headaches, constipation, itching with no rash (especially at night)? Do you swell more as the day goes on? Do you develop cysts easily? Do you break out in skin rashes or have skin sensitivity? Are you chemically sensitive? All of these are signs to me that you probably have a toxic body.

When the body is not able to cleanse out waste material or toxins properly or efficiently, the body can become overworked and overloaded with toxins. Sometimes we need to do things to help our body clean out the toxins. It is my opinion that until we get rid of the toxic body, until we remove the sources and cleanse out the toxins, the environment of our bodies will be ideal for bacteria and fungus to thrive and infections will continue. You can take antibiotics and/or antifungals (natural or synthetic) over and over again, but the infections will keep coming back. Cysts and tumors will develop more easily and readily in a toxic body. As long as the body remains toxic, we will continue to develop all kinds of allergies and sensitivities to foods, vitamins, chemicals, and various things in the environment. But we have to start somewhere. And it is wise to start where you are.

This is a very important step, not only because it is where we begin to determine our path, but also because it is something we need to do all the time. We need to continually re-evaluate where we are in the moment and make adjustments to what we're doing based on how we are feeling.

Part of determining your present situation is in Steps 4 and 5.

Step 4 - Identify your allergies/sensitivities

Medically speaking, it is fairly well known that IC patients often have allergies and sensitivities. If we didn't have them before IC, we often develop them after we get IC. There are some allergies that we might be aware of and some that maybe we aren't. And even if we are aware of our allergies, what can we do about it? When I became chemically sensitive with my IC and developed countless allergies, it was not as simple as avoiding allergens or taking an antihistamine. Allergies are not always just a stuffy nose and watery eyes like you see on the commercials. An allergic reaction can come in many forms. For me, I eventually discovered that various allergies I had caused swelling all over my body, mysterious skin rashes, difficulty breathing, an increase in bladder symptoms, IBS symptoms, fibro symptoms, Vulvodynia symptoms, and (just in case I wasn't having enough fun) sometimes my throat would close up making it difficult to swallow and breath. I was not able to go anywhere or be near people. Nearly everything set off a reaction in my body and bladder. Perfume, cigarette smoke, exhaust fumes, paint fumes, new carpeting, hairsprays, detergents, chemical cleaners, they all made me sick to be around. Anything chemical or toxic was the worst, but even foods and natural things could cause me to have a reaction. And the scariest part of all was that I could develop a new allergy at any time. Something I could have eaten or taken for a long time and had no problem with, could all of a sudden one day cause a horrible allergic reaction. Knowing what I was allergic to was only part of it. And usually I didn't know. Then for the allergens I did figure out, avoiding them seemed near impossible. Actually it didn't seem impossible. It *was* impossible. I honestly don't know what I would have done had I not found an answer to this problem through NAET.

NAET is an allergy elimination technique that uses acupuncture and/or acupressure along with kinesiology in order to identify and eliminate allergies. NAET stands for Nambudripad Allergy Elimination Technique. (Dr. Devi Nambudripad, author of the book "Say Goodbye to Illness", invented the technique.) After determining what you are allergic to, you are put in contact with the allergen during treatment. Then, by opening up the energy pathways of the body (meridians) using acupuncture and/or acupressure, NAET retrains the body (and the central nervous system) to "accept" the presence of the allergen instead of viewing it as an "enemy". After a 24-25 hour avoidance period, you are re-introduced to the allergen purposely in order to (confirm) the treatment. From then on, your allergy is gone. (I was cleared for a total of 41 allergies in the end. It has been well over a year and a half since my last treatment and none of my allergies have returned. However, I do feel that if I would have remained toxic (i.e., not removed my fillings and cleansed out the mercury or not quit smoking for example) that I would probably have seen some of my allergies return. In other words, NAET worked great, but I definitely had to do other things as well in order to get better.)

As I said in *To Wake In Tears*, I think NAET is a great treatment option for IC patients for several reasons. First of all, it is painless, non-invasive, and you don't have to ingest anything. All three of those things make it more likely that an IC patient can tolerate the treatments. It allows the IC patient to overcome vitamin and food sensitivities which enable the person to be able to eat things they couldn't eat before, take vitamin and/or herbal supplements that they couldn't tolerate before, and have a better chance to get the nutrition needed to help their body and bladder to heal. I believe this is a very important side benefit of NAET for IC patients. NAET also helps tremendously just in the fact that it quickly and painlessly identifies exactly what we are allergic to. This is all not to mention that NAET is great for IC patients because it actually works and eliminates allergies.

During NAET treatments, I would recommend doing soothing things at the same time, getting lots of rest, and drinking lots of water. I remember I took a lot of acidophilus and drank marshmallow root tea to support and soothe my bladder and intestines through the cleansing that occurs from the NAET. I wouldn't advise taking anything orally that is cleansing during this time (especially for those with more severe IC) because the NAET will already be doing enough cleansing. At the same time, if you are having your fillings replaced at the same time that you are doing NAET, then I would maybe do one other mild thing to help cleanse (like Colostrum for example). Actually I would recommend having your fillings replaced once you are already doing NAET for a couple reasons. You would then have the opportunity to be tested and treated for a mercury allergy prior to having the dental work done. This way you would help minimize the negative effects during and after removal. Also, if you finish the NAET treatments and rid yourself of your allergies and then decide to have your fillings replaced, you will run the risk, in my opinion, that it will stir everything up again and then some of your allergies might come back. You may then need to go back to have a few follow up NAET treatments.

I always remind my IC friends to take all of their medications, herbs, or whatever they're taking or planning to take every day, to their NAET doctor so they can be tested. Just to make sure that what they are taking is helping, rather than hurting them. This can be a tremendous help. You can be taking something for a long time and it can be helping you. But then something mysterious happens and our bodies build up a resistance to it or sensitivity to it and we don't even realize it. I know this happened to me with several things. Aloe vera is a good example. I drank aloe vera juice for a while to help soothe my intestines and bladder. I did great with it for a while, but then something in me said not to drink it anymore even though I wasn't sure if it was bothering me or not. I listened to my gut and stopped drinking it. (Plus I hated the taste...hee!) Anyway, a few months later when I started NAET, I discovered I was allergic to aloe. And I had been using aloe vera toilet paper too! I had no idea I was allergic to it. It turned out that my Vulvodynia symptoms improved greatly after being treated for aloe. I actually brought in a sample of the toilet paper and was treated for aloe and the aloe toilet paper at the same time. If you have Vulvodynia and you're going to NAET, I would take a sample of your toilet paper to be tested for. Even the fabric of your underwear, the detergent you wash your underwear with, and your own urine. They can all be causing an allergic reaction and I would suggest getting tested for them. In fact, I think it would be really interesting to have all IC patients tested to see if they are allergic to their own urine. According to NAET doctors, we can be allergic to our own blood, our partners' semen, even our own saliva. All of our bodily fluids can be tested and treated for.

In terms of being able to tolerate the treatments bladder-wise, I would say that it's wise to have your bladder in decent shape. In other words, I know that I could never have tolerated having the NAET treatments back when my bladder was still bleeding. Ironically, the reason for this is actually another reason why I think NAET is great for IC patients. It is because NAET also helps to re-balance and cleanse the body. This is a really good thing, but you have to be ready for it. Your bladder has to be able to handle the extra toxins being passed through the urine. Your body, and you, have to be ready for your symptoms to change and for you to maybe get a little worse before you get better (which is what typically happens whenever you cleanse). It takes patience and courage to go through NAET treatments because there are a lot of changes that occur along the way. If you're bladder isn't in good enough shape to tolerate the treatments right now, you can at least get muscle tested for your allergies to find out whether what you are taking (or intending on taking) is something you're allergic to or not.

NAET is a mild cleanse in terms of the fact that you don't have to ingest anything, but it can definitely produce strong cleansing symptoms and/or increase your symptoms for a time as your body is re-balancing. The more toxic you are, the more cleansing symptoms you might have and/or the more severe your cleansing symptoms might be. Also remember that the effects of the treatments are not just for one or two days. It takes time after each treatment for the body to cleanse and re-balance so you will see effects of the treatments in terms of symptoms changes for some time (e.g., weeks and sometimes months). This is all a good thing and you will be able to tell that you are getting better and stronger, etc. At the same time, it can be scary when our symptoms get worse for a day or two; or when one thing gets better, but then another thing gets worse. But like I said, all in all we can usually tell that we are getting better. This is the confusing thing about doing anything that cleanses the body and I will talk more about this in Step 6.

If you're not planning to take antibiotics for your IC and are aware that you do have allergies, to me this is a really good beginning step (along with soothing your bladder of course). After you get yourself out of pain and as long as your bladder is not bleeding badly, I think it's great to find an NAET doctor as soon as you can. If for no other reason than to find out exactly what you're allergic to. This way you can make sure that the things that you are taking to help you are actually helping, rather than hurting you. I think this is a very important step in the right direction. And if you can tolerate it, and at the pace you can afford to do it (because for some people it might not be covered by your insurance), you will be able to start eliminating your allergies and slowly getting your body back into balance.

What if you can't find an NAET doctor? Or what if you can't afford the treatments because they aren't covered by your insurance? Or maybe you simply don't believe something like this would work for you. How else can you determine your allergies? You could go to an allergist and have an Elisa/Act allergy test done to find out what you're allergic to. If trying an herb or natural product, you could always put a little bit on your tongue first and see if you have a reaction before trying it. Or at the worst, you'd be stuck with the old trial and error method that most people have probably used thus far. Just remember to use as small an amount as possible your first time. Sometimes the only way to know for sure is to give it a shot. Lastly, you could learn to muscle test yourself at home to check for allergies the same way the NAET doctor would do it. If you get the book *Say Goodbye to Illness* by Dr. Devi Nambudripad who invented NAET, you can read about how to do it yourself at home. Or you could go to one or two NAET appointments and learn how to test yourself at home. It's a very quick and easy thing to do once you know how.

Step 5 - Identify your sources of toxins and eliminate them as much as possible

As I was discussing earlier, there are many sources of toxins that can be affecting you. The trick is to determine where your sources of toxins are coming from and then the even bigger trick is trying to eliminate them. It would be helpful to make a list of all the possible sources of toxins that might be affecting you so that you'll know where to start. For me it was cigarette smoke, candida, food and environmental allergies, medications that I took when I was first sick, and last, but certainly not least, were my mercury amalgam fillings. Remember that stress causes toxins in the body. And as you know, stress is not an easy thing to get rid of, but we have to do our best to eliminate it as much as possible. Knowing that stress is inhibiting us from getting better and is possibly making us worse, we might have to ask for help from our loved ones in order to be able to reduce our stress level. Actually, this is something we need to consider with ALL of our sources, that they could possibly be inhibiting us from getting better and that they could be making us worse. If you have tried many approaches to getting better and nothing seems to be helping...or if you've tried things that have helped for a time, but then they stopped helping, and you seem to be getting even worse...I would look to your list of "sources" to see what might be inhibiting you.

Though this list is by no means exhaustive, the following are all possible sources of toxins that you might want to consider.

Stress
Mercury amalgam fillings
Chronic constipation
Candida (yeast) overgrowth
Food allergies
Environmental allergies
Pharmaceutical medications
Artificial sweeteners and other chemical food additives
Exposure to chemicals, metals, or synthetics
Cigarette smoke
Alcohol
Caffeine

You might want to sit down with yourself and/or your loved ones and determine what is draining your energy; what exactly is stressing you, both emotionally and physically. You might need to make some tough decisions about how to eliminate these things to the best of your ability, even if only temporarily while you are healing. Once you are well, you will be able to handle more stress than you can right now. Stress, right now, is only going to make you worse and make it harder for you to heal. But I don't have to tell you that. I know that you already know that. The thing is, most of the time, we have trouble realizing that we can control any of it. Asking for help in eliminating stress, as well as providing that comfort for yourself are two very difficult things for people to do. But know this for certain. If you are intending to heal from IC and all of it's related symptoms/illnesses, eliminating stress in your life, eliminating toxic relationships and people who are not supportive of you or who may, intentionally or unintentionally, be emotionally or verbally abusive to you is very important. In fact, it is my opinion that these things are crucial. It will be very difficult for you to heal in an environment that is completely unsupportive of you loving yourself and taking care of yourself. Making the necessary changes in order to help our bodies heal is just one of the things that's a total pain in the neck about getting better. Eliminating (or at least reducing) stress is *not* going to be easy. And eliminating the other toxins that are affecting you probably won't be too easy either. Okay now that I've cheered you up, let's talk about some other sources of toxins that are, in my opinion, crucial to get rid of in order to heal.

Some of the things on the list of sources are obviously poisons to our body, while others are less accepted as being harmful. For example, cigarettes are obviously full of chemicals and poisons. Most people know about that. We have known for years that they are bad for us and it's only gotten worse as they changed the ingredients over the years. Stress and/or constipation are sources of toxins to our body that we don't generally think about in that way. And then there is systemic candida, which is not even accepted as "an issue" by most AMA doctors. Just as mercury amalgam fillings are said to be safe by ADA dentists. Or that aspartame is considered safe because it is "FDA approved". Learning more about these chemicals that are being put into our foods and drinks, learning more about the metals that they are putting into our mouths, learning more about the chemicals we are smoking or ingesting through pharmaceuticals, just looking into them further is what I'm suggesting here. Read about them and learn more about what they might be doing to your body. If you take the time, I'm sure you will be as horrified as I was to find out what all of these things are known to do, what they are *proven* to cause, and what they are probably doing to you.

Remember we are typically more sensitive than people who don't have IC. We are known to develop multiple allergies and to be more sensitive to things in general. The more severe your IC, the more likely you are to be extra sensitive. Some of us have sensitive skin; some are sensitive to light, to loud noises, to all kinds of smells, to all kinds of foods, to vitamins, to minerals, to nearly everything. So when you're reading more about these various sources, I would keep that in mind. A question I get fairly often is "what if I only have one or two "silver" fillings? Do you think they could be causing a problem?" Well first of all, I can't tell you that because we are all different. But I can tell you that if I were you, I'd have them replaced. What I can tell you is that it only takes one filling to cause a problem, especially if you are allergic to or sensitive to the metals used in fillings. (Since the 70's, mercury amalgam fillings contain 50% mercury, 35% silver, 9% tin, 6% copper, and a trace of zinc.) The way I look at it, if you're sensitive to many things and especially if your sensitive to nearly everything, foods and natural things that normally don't hurt people, why would you think you wouldn't be sensitive to something that is a known poison? This would be my perspective. Granted, I am biased because my fillings were definitely a huge factor in the toxicity of my body. I know for certain that I would not be better today had I not had them removed. But that was just my experience. It doesn't mean it will be yours.

So how do you know if your fillings are affecting you? First of all, there are tests that you can have done to check for mercury (and other heavy metal) toxicity. You can have a hair analysis, urine analysis, blood test, or even be checked via NAET to find out if you're allergic/sensitive to it. Just remember, you can be tested with NAET and found to be not allergic to mercury, but that doesn't necessarily mean that it's not causing you any problems. It just means you're not allergic to it. No matter what, it's a poison and our body views it that way automatically. It's really a matter of whether you are processing it

53

out of you efficiently. For those people who are healthy, who exercise regularly, who aren't extra sensitive, and who have the vitamins and minerals in their body to help process the mercury, their fillings probably won't be as big of a deal for them. Not everyone is going to be negatively affected by their fillings (obviously). I just feel that IC patients will be more likely than "regular" people to be affected by them. For one thing, we often have a weakened immune system, we often are more sensitive as I've mentioned, we often are lacking in certain key vitamins and minerals that our body needs to process these types of things, and lastly, we are often experiencing symptoms that are common with mercury poisoning. The following are some questions that you can ask yourself to help you determine whether your "silver" fillings are affecting you. Do you have jaw pain or TMJ, earaches, and/or sore throats all the time? Have you been told that you grind your teeth? Do you have a metal taste in your mouth? Are you super insanely sensitive to smells, especially perfumes, exhaust fumes, paint fumes, and other synthetic chemical smells? Do you have sinus problems? Do you have a coated tongue? Do you have receding gums? Are your teeth chipping or moving around (shifting) in your mouth? Do you have blisters and/or canker sores in your mouth or throat? Do you have inflamed gums and sensitive teeth? These are all red flags to me that mercury might be an issue for you. If you answered yes to several of these questions, I would definitely read more about mercury amalgam fillings.

Now just because you get your fillings replaced does not mean you will automatically solve all your health problems. More must be done to get better. Cleansing out the mercury that has been stored in your body is one very important thing. I know some people who have had their fillings replaced, but didn't do anything to cleanse afterward. Most likely they didn't see much of a health improvement from the removal because the mercury has remained in the tissues of the body. Also, mercury will not necessarily be your only source of toxins. For me, it was huge, yes. But it certainly wasn't the only thing. I know other people who have had their fillings replaced, but they still smoke, for example. Your other sources will continue to cause your body to be toxic and if you add that to not cleansing out the mercury after removal, it is logical to me that you wouldn't see as much of a health improvement. And lastly, if you have had your fillings replaced and didn't see much of a health improvement or haven't noticed anything yet it could be that it hasn't been that long of a period of time to be able to notice anything or that maybe it wasn't a huge source of poison to your body. Maybe there are other sources that are affecting you still or maybe there are other sources that are affecting you more. We are not all going to be the same (as usual).

One last thing I wanted to mention on this subject is that I also know IC patients who have had some of their fillings replaced and have stopped in the middle because they feel like they are getting worse. They feel the extra sensitivity in the teeth, even more so now than before they started having them replaced. This can happen and did happen to me as well. In the midst of having them replaced, my teeth did become more sensitive and things did get worse for a while before they got better. There was all that poison to process through my body as it started clearing out of my gums. It's just like when you quit smoking and your immune system starts to kick in and start cleansing out the poisons. It makes you sick. This is the same thing. And our teeth can get extra sensitive because the nerves are getting even more irritated while the poisons are working their way out and it takes time for the nerves to heal. If you are in this situation, all I can tell you is that if I were in your shoes, I would finish getting them all done. It takes time after having them all out for your whole mouth to heal, for your whole body to heal really. It doesn't happen overnight. I remember hearing that when you quit smoking it takes seven years for your lungs to clean out. I don't know if that's totally accurate or anything, but I do know that it takes time to get better regardless of what sources you're removing.

As important as the next two steps are, if you don't identify and eliminate the sources of toxins to your body, in my opinion, you will either have to continually cleanse and/or you will continue to be sick. I **feel it is crucial to get rid of the sources.** And I'll tell you...this is NOT news I want to deliver. This is not news anyone wants to hear. I know that. And I know that certainly I wouldn't have wanted anyone telling me that I might need to quit smoking or maybe I wouldn't get better. (In fact, my mom did tell me that and naturally I was totally annoyed with her and didn't want to listen.) Or that maybe it would be wise to go to the dentist (where I totally hated going) and think about having all my fillings replaced! I don't know that I would have listened for one minute to someone who was telling me that my teeth had anything at all to do with my bladder symptoms or my health. I didn't want to hear about mercury being a poison. I didn't want to spend the money or the time going to the dentist over something that may or may not have anything to do with my health problems. And besides, isn't almost everyone exposed to these things all the time and they don't all have IC. I probably would have thought they were nuts. As crazy as it may sound (and I know to some people it might sound crazy), I will tell you now what I tell IC patients that I talk to all the time. I know for certain (as certain as a person can know anything) that I would NOT be better today had I not had my mercury fillings replaced, quit smoking, reduced my stress, and changed my eating habits to more nutritious, non-chemical foods. I am not saying that these things alone are what got me better. It took MUCH more than that. But what I am saying is that I could have done all the other stuff I did (NAET, herbs, candida cleanse, etc.), but if I hadn't removed the sources of poison to my body, I would not be better today. As I tell my IC friends...I could have cleansed till the cows came home and I would still be sick. I could have drank marshmallow root tea for the rest of my life and gone to NAET religiously and I would still not be better. I could have followed an IC diet, anti-candida diet, or low oxalate diet the rest of my life, but it would not have gotten me better. I could have soothed my bladder, boosted my immune system, and exercised consistently and although all of these things are great things to do, I would *still* not be better had I not removed the major sources of poison to my body. I cannot stress this enough. If you get anything at all from this book, I hope you get this point because it will take you farther in terms of getting better than anything else. If the sources of toxins to your body are not removed, it will be near impossible to get better. (In my opinion of course.) Yes you can get somewhat better. And yes you can improve by doing these other things. You can maybe even get yourself into remission. But if you want to get better all the way. If you want to return your bladder and body to a state of normal health, where you can eat what you want, have sex with no pain, heck, live with no pain or bladder symptoms of any kind, and be, you know, NORMAL...then you HAVE to remove the sources.

Please also keep in mind that I did not get rid of any of my sources of toxins overnight. And personally, I don't think it's wise to do it all at once and I'll tell you why. **With each source of toxin that you remove, your body will automatically start cleansing itself.** I wrote about this in *To Wake In Tears*; about how when I quit smoking, I got very sick. I had no idea that when I quit smoking, my body would react that way. I had no idea that there was even the *possibility* that quitting smoking would make me sick. But what I learned was that as soon as you remove a source of poison to the body, your immune system will automatically start kicking in and will be trying to cleanse the poisons out. This can cause a variety of symptoms depending on the person. For me, when I quit smoking, I got a huge horrible flu/cold with horrible chest congestion where I could barely breathe. It was very scary and very unexpected by me. I thought I'd start feeling better from quitting smoking, not get worse! This is also a good example of how sometimes we seem to get worse before we can get better. It is this way whenever you remove a source of poison to the body. With each source you remove, with each filling you get replaced, with each food or allergen that you start to avoid (or get cleared through NAET), with each medication you stop taking, your body will automatically start to cleanse itself. We can also do things to help our body cleanse the bad stuff out, which leads us to Step 6.

Step 6 - Cleanse gently and slowly

Cleansing the body, as well as the knowledge of the importance of doing so, has been around for centuries. This is not a new concept I'm talking about here. The main difference is that with IC, there are many more things to be careful of when cleansing. If you read about cleansing, you will probably come across cleansing diets, juice cleanses, fasting cleanses, herbal cleanses, and even things like homeopathic cleanses, enemas, colonics, and chelation therapy. Most of these types of cleanses, I believe, are way too strong for someone who has IC, especially someone who has a moderate to severe case of IC. When it comes to IC, it is my opinion that the most important thing is to cleanse GENTLY and SLOWLY. If you go too fast, you will make yourself much more sick in the process. We are much more toxic than an ordinary person (or even someone with another illness) that might want to do some cleansing. Our bladders are only going to be able to take so much. Certain types of cleanses are going to be major no-no's for an IC patient. De-tox tea at the health food store, for example, is going to be way too strong for most IC patients. Cleansing with juices or apple cider vinegar is obviously not the way to go if you have IC. Neither are many of the herbal cleanses that are on the market. Many of them contain combinations of herbs and in my opinion are going to be much too strong for someone with IC. We are fortunate that nature provides us with many gentle alternatives, as you will see in the next couple sections of this book. But first...

What does it mean to cleanse? And how do you know when you are cleansing? There are many forms of cleansing. Some are natural (they occur whether we do anything specific or not) and others are induced either by natural or synthetic means. There are many herbs and natural products that are cleansing to the body. And although many people probably don't think of it that way, even Diflucan (a prescription anti-fungal medication) is cleansing to the body. A woman's menstrual cycle is a good example of a natural cleanse. There are also certain foods that are just naturally cleansing to the body. Garlic and onions are good examples. Whenever you are doing anything that re-balances the body, such as NAET, acupuncture, acupressure, even reflexology and massage, they are all cleansing to the body. Anything that helps move the lymph system and/or breaks up toxins will help cleanse the body. Exercise is another good example of something that causes a natural cleanse. Herbal baths can also be cleansing. I'll be expanding on all of these things more in Section 6.

A healing reaction or cleansing reaction occurs because the body is ridding itself of the substances that have been making it toxic. It is caused by the flushing of toxins out of the cells and tissues, and then out of the body. As these substances are cleansed from the cells and tissues, they are first dumped into our system, which makes the body temporarily even more toxic until the substances can be excreted. This is partly what produces the symptoms of the healing reaction. It is also caused by the body tearing apart defective tissues, repairing damaged cells, destroying infections like bacteria, fungi, and parasites and ridding itself of the other debris from the rebuilding. The more severe your IC, the more toxic your body, the stronger the healing reaction will be. So you'll have to be prepared that you might appear to get worse before you start to get better. This is a normal part of the healing process and yes, it totally happened that way for me too of course. Often we will re-experience old symptoms that will return temporarily on our way back to health. It's very difficult not to be alarmed when this happens. This is the part where it's hard to hang in there. It's hard to wait it out and allow our bodies to go through what they need to go through in order to cleanse and heal itself. If we panic and take medications to cover the symptoms, we will be putting a stop to (or at the very least) slowing down the cleansing and healing process.

When you cleanse, certain symptoms typically appear. You might get headaches, diarrhea, vaginal discharge, and an increase in bladder symptoms due to the toxins leaving your body through the urine. You might also get an increase in Vulvodynia symptoms due to the discharge and increased toxicity of your urine. You might feel even more fatigued, more sore and achy all over. (At this point you're probably thinking okay...now WHY did I decide to cleanse?) You might get skin rashes and/or skin itching and inflammation, increased mucous (again, worse than usual) whether through the stools, the sinuses, the lungs, or through vaginal discharge, increased body odor, sweating and/or feelings of being flushed, and stronger urine odor and

59

stool odor as more toxins/poisons leave your system. In other words, you may feel an increase in all of your symptoms for a time. This is why I always say that it's so hard to know if what you're doing is a good thing or a bad thing. In other words, are you having a "reaction" to the herbs or whatever you're taking or are you "just" cleansing? Are you getting worse or getting better? Sometimes it's really hard to tell. But just in recognizing all the different types of things that can cause your body to cleanse and knowing what symptoms typically occur FOR YOU when you're cleansing, it will make it easier for you to know as time goes on. You will be able to recognize the fact that you are either taking something or doing something (or for natural reasons) and that your body is cleansing itself. How long this increase in symptoms or cleansing reaction will last will be different for everyone based on how toxic you are, how fast you are removing your sources, and how fast you are cleansing.

As you cleanse, toxins will be released through all the eliminative channels and your urine, among other things, will become more toxic. This is why it is so important to soothe while you are doing anything or taking anything that is cleansing to the body. It is so important for an IC patient to support their bladder and kidneys throughout the cleansing process. It is also important to support your intestines by replacing friendly bacteria (acidophilus/probiotics) and the rest of the body as well by taking as good care of yourself as you possibly can. Getting as much rest as possible and significantly reducing your stress level are both very important. As you cleanse, toxins will also be released through your skin since it is the largest eliminative organ. This is why I think it's important and helpful to take healing baths or to do some skin brushing. (See section 6) This will help support the release of toxins through your skin.

So let's say you decide that you are toxic and that you do think you need to cleanse your body. How do you decide what to do? First I'd keep the following in mind. With each source of toxin you remove, your body will automatically be cleansing itself. In other words, you need not necessarily TAKE anything and your body will already be cleansing.

However, usually we need to do more than simply remove the source. But it's still important to remember that this happens. Not only because you will end up seeing cleansing symptoms whenever you remove a source, but also because you don't want to do too many cleansing things at the same time. If you do some form of exercise on a regular basis or use acupressure, acupuncture, NAET, reflexology, or any form of massage, your body will automatically be cleansing itself. If you drink plenty of water (which is highly recommended when you have IC), the water will be gently and naturally flushing your body. If you have trouble ingesting things because you are very sensitive, I would consider starting with some of the things listed in Section 6 of this book. If you feel you have a problem with yeast (candida) I would consider starting with some type of candida cleanse. (This was really where I first started consciously cleansing.) Most people recommend first cleansing the colon and then going from there, even if you don't necessarily have a yeast problem. This is also what I would recommend. You wouldn't want to go right into a liver or lymphatic cleanse for example. That would be WAY too harsh for someone with IC in my opinion. I made that mistake myself and have seen others make it as well. We were all told by alternative health practitioners of some sort that we had a toxic liver and our lymph glands needed cleansing. All of this was very true. BUT, the problem is that these cleanses are extremely strong for someone who has a very toxic body and is ultra sensitive. All this approach will do is make a person with IC much worse.

When reading through the herbs and natural products (sections 4 and 5) you can make a list of some of the cleansing things you might want to look into further. When you start looking for cleansing herbs or natural products, just remember that you don't want to take too many cleansing things at once or DO too many cleansing things at once either. I think one thing that helped me get better was that I basically only ingested one cleansing thing at a time. Cleansing too fast is something you do not want to do when you have IC. If you cleanse too fast or too hard you will definitely feel it. You will definitely be able to tell. It's so important to be gentle and to go slow. It's a process that's not going to happen over night. But at least you know you are heading in the right direction even though you might not feel so good along the way. It's very helpful to pay attention to and keep track of how you are feeling and then to go with what your body is telling you. We will all be different (what else is new), so you can't always go by what happens to someone else.

You can also over-cleanse and cause yourself even more problems. If you cleanse too long or too hard you can get too low on electrolytes and nutrients and then you can get sick in other ways. This brings me to the last major step in recovering from IC.

Step 7 - Rebuilding

It is so hugely important to rebuild after cleansing. Rebuilding is something we often forget. We think of cleansing out the bad, but we sometimes forget about rebuilding the good. This is something you hear often with candida cleansing programs. After a candida cleanse, it is highly recommended to take LOTS of acidophilus in order to replace the friendly bacteria in the intestines. And just as we need to replace the friendly bacteria to bring the intestinal flora back into balance, we also need to replace nutrients, vitamins, minerals, enzymes, and amino acids for example, to bring our body back into balance after cleansing. This is another reason I feel NAET is extremely helpful for IC patients. It can enable us to be able to take vitamins, minerals, and other things needed to help us rebuild and replenish our bodies so that our bodies and bladder can heal all the way.

With IC we are so toxic that it is not necessarily going to be enough to do a candida cleanse or to simply remove the sources of toxins. Well actually, I take that back. For some people who have mild IC, it might be. But for those of us with more severe IC, we might find ourselves having to cleanse for long periods or cleanse in different ways. Remember, it is good to take breaks from cleansing so that you can rebuild. Or you can even do some rebuilding while you're cleansing because your cleansing period might be fairly long in duration. I did both. I sometimes took a break from cleansing and I also did things to replenish my body during cleansing. Because our cleansing period might be several weeks or months for example, it's important to be rebuilding along the way. This is so important so that you don't strip your body of all its needed nutrients and electrolytes, which, by the way, you are probably lacking to begin with. If you over-cleanse without doing some rebuilding, you will cause yourself to develop new and different symptoms.

Rebuilding is also important to do if your bladder and body are torn down right now. If that is the case for you, as I said earlier, you might want to do this step first along with soothing your bladder and getting yourself out of pain. The problem will be HOW to get this extra nutrition into your body. When my IC was really bad and I was extremely bloated, I found it very difficult to eat. Not only was I limited in my food choices based on what I could tolerate bladder-wise, but I was also limited because the more I ate, the worse I usually felt. All the extra pressure from a full stomach made me feel worse and digestion was difficult and very uncomfortable. I usually could only eat one decent meal a day and that was dinner. I would wait until Charlie was home with me because I knew I was going to feel worse. I was losing a lot of weight and I don't think I was absorbing much nutrition from the food I was able to eat. I found that some type of nutrition drink works best at this point. Just in the fact that it is liquid and is easier to digest and absorb is very helpful. Finding a good nutrition drink that you can tolerate takes some effort, but health food stores usually have many choices. I drank an herbal rebuilder drink from Hannah Kroger that I thought worked great and it was very mellow on the bladder. Later when my bladder was in much better shape, I drank Ensure's with a banana, liquid acidophilus, yogurt, a crushed up amino acid pill, a couple drops of liquid minerals, and Glucosamine sulfate (because my fibro was bad at that point). With a little creativity and a blender, you will be able to find a nutrition drink of your own that works for you. The main thing is to get as much easily absorbable nutrition into your body

63

as you possibly can without irritating your bladder. Rebuilding and bringing balance back to your body is as important as cleansing out the toxins. If you get through some cleansing and you aren't sure what you need to take to help your body rebalance, it can be helpful to have some tests done to find out. You can have blood tests done to measure vitamin and mineral deficiencies and this will help you figure out what you need to rebuild your body.

At this point, you will have a list of affected organs (along with your symptoms), a list of possible sources of toxins to your body, and a list of where you are in the moment, or rather, a "possible things to consider" list. For example, yours might say things like, send a sample to Dr. Fugazzotto, read more about systemic candida or find a way to get tested for candida, read more about the toxic body or get tested for mercury and heavy metals. You may have decided that you're in a torn down stage right now and need to soothe and rebuild versus jumping right into cleansing. You might have decided that your symptoms are most likely allergy driven and maybe checking out NAET doctors in your area might be on your list. You will also be able to make a list of possible options to cleanse your body, as well as possible options to soothe your bladder (stomach, intestines, etc.) by reading through the herbs and natural products in sections 4 and 5. You might decide that you are just way too sensitive right now to be able to tolerate any of these herbs and instead you might want to look at some of the options in section 6 under "Things you don't have to ingest". You will be able to take your list of affected organs (and symptoms) and look for natural, non-toxic things to soothe and support those organs. You'll be able to take a look at your list of possible sources of toxins and decide when and how you want to remove those sources. It might be as simple as no longer drinking diet soda and avoiding certain allergens or it might be as complicated as having to quit smoking, replace your fillings, quit your job that is around chemicals, or deciding whether to continue on with your pharmaceutical medications. It might even involve getting away from what I call toxic relationships or toxic situations in your life that cause you a lot of stress. It is difficult to heal when you're in these situations and it will be up to you to decide if you can. It will be up to you to make yourself a priority, to make your healing a priority.

Section 3

Stones Along the Path

As you struggle to get better (hey…I never said it was easy), there are problems you may run into, setbacks that might occur, and questions that might come up. You might wonder if you're on the right track or not with your treatment. More than that, you might be totally scared and wondering if you're doing the right thing. This is all very normal. I was scared most of the time that I was getting better. All right, forget "most". I think I was scared the entire time. There are so many scary things about having IC. Though, if you have IC, I don't have to tell you that. There are risks with all of the available treatments and medications. There are risks with "alternative" treatments and medical treatments alike. There are no easy answers and no sure fire treatment, so it can be very confusing for us to know what to do. I'm not sure which is scarier, going the medical route or going the natural route. I suppose they both have scary things about them. Well, at least to me they do.

Some people feel that it's safer to go the medical route because at least then you have a doctor advising you on what to take and how much, advising you on what treatment to try next, etc. And I can certainly understand why they would feel that way. At the same time, there are other people who don't feel safe at all about going to a urologist for their IC. I know several IC patients who don't go to a urologist. And though there are scary things about going the natural approach, some people feel that the medical treatments currently being offered are either painful and invasive or carry risks of short and long-term side effects. Some people don't feel comfortable with the approach of trying to cover up symptoms and then learning to live with it. Others feel that they have no other choice and until the medical community discovers a cure, they are stuck with IC and must do what the doctor advises. They feel this is the only wise course of action and may even be horrified at the thought of not going to a urologist for their IC. We are all different in how we feel about these issues and we all need to do what makes us feel the least afraid, the most safe, and the most comfortable.

I can understand why some people feel safer taking only things that are recommended by their physician. At the same time, I would still strongly encourage people to do research on their own even after getting their physician's recommendation. There is nothing wrong with researching things on your own just to make sure. And though I can understand the fear that some people have about taking herbs or natural products that are not recommended by their doctor, at the same time I can also understand why some people are afraid of taking prescribed synthetic medications as well. Both have risks. Both you need to be careful with. And yet both have their place in helping us heal (if you ask me anyway).

As I discuss the good and the bad of both the medical community and the "naturals" or "alternatives" as I will call them, I must tell you this. I have been hurt by both: by both medical doctors and "natural" or "alternative" doctors, by healers and herbologists alike. I admit, as I write this, that I must temper my bias toward either side for their faults/mistakes. Medical doctors and alternative healers/practitioners, they are all doing the best they can. They are almost always trying to help (well...except for the idiots who don't think IC exists), but they just don't understand. I don't believe they understand the magnitude of how IC affects the rest of the body. And, most importantly, I don't believe they understand how much harm they can cause without realizing it. As I write this, I must remind myself, and you (all of you who have been hurt like me), that they are all just doing the best they can. And that we, the IC patients, just need to be aware. We need to remember that they are just people doing the best they can with a disease that they don't fully understand. And most importantly, we need to make sure that we protect ourselves. We need to read and research much more than a sick person would ever want to. We need to make sure to remember that when we walk out that door, when we leave that doctor's office (medical or natural), we are on our own. We are the ones who have to live with the consequences of the things they want us to try. We need to recognize when we are trusting our health to a professional person who may or may not have the time to stay up on the latest IC research. We need to recognize when we are trusting our doctor to understand, not only IC in general, but OUR IC (because we're all different). And then, not only OUR IC, but also what is best for our whole body. Does your doctor take that much time with you? If he/she does, you are VERY lucky indeed.

Alternative or medical, it's very rare to come across a professional health care provider that is going to understand YOUR IC enough, know your body well enough, to know what is best for you to do and for you to take. This is why the responsibility is ours. In my opinion, no matter how you look at, unless you are among the extremely fortunate, WE are ultimately responsible. Everyone in our society always wants to make the doctor responsible. "Check with your doctor", we hear it every day all over the place. People will say this or that and always add, "check with your doctor". This takes the responsibility off of them for saying whatever it is they are saying, and puts it on the doctor. It takes the responsibility away from the individual for his or her own health and puts it on their doctor instead. Our doctors (medical or natural) are not gods. No matter how wonderful and well trained, no matter what good grades they got in medical school or how wonderful a bedside manner, they are not perfect. And we have to recognize that and not expect or even hope that they are going to have all the answers for us. We have to find our own answers based on our own individual situations and based on our own research into what we feel most comfortable doing to our bodies. In the end, we have to be responsible.

We need to remember, medical or natural, layperson or "IC expert", that not much has been proven yet when it comes to IC and that how we are being treated is based on that particular person or doctor's perspective/opinion of what IC is. Most urologists will treat as if IC is only in the bladder. Some natural or alternative doctors will treat as if IC is a systemic infection, whether bacterial, viral, or fungal. Some will treat as if it's a muscle problem (i.e., pelvic floor dysfunction or PFD) or a nerve problem. Some will treat as if it's a back problem or a hormone problem. We need to keep in mind that how we are being treated is based on what that doctor or person thinks IC is all about. We need to decide what WE think IC is (at least for us) and then hopefully find a doctor who's coming from that same perspective.

If you are going to someone who is supposedly an "IC expert", please remember to ask what kind of research he/she is doing. Please make sure you are not just another number in their study. I know this sounds harsh, but I've seen it happen often. If your doctor commands you to follow his/her treatment protocol and you don't feel it is right for you, please find another doctor. This happened to me and many other people I know. My first urologist appointment after being diagnosed with severe IC, the doctor told me he wanted to do bladder instillations. I told him how I had met a lot of IC patients on line and learned that there were other options that I wanted to try first, less invasive options. He told me, "no bladder instillations, no pain medication". He told me that this was his treatment protocol; this was the way *he* treated IC. And then went on to tell me that I must not be in enough pain or I would do the instillations. This was from the "IC expert" in the city where I live. Now, I'm aware that some people might be thinking, oh well this guy was a jerk then, but this is probably an exception. Well…no. I'm afraid it's not. It happens a lot. It's not easy to find a good doctor when you have IC. A doctor (alternative or medical) should not "command" you do to anything. Suggest maybe. Advise maybe. But not command, or else. In other words, do this or I won't treat you.

I encourage you to keep looking if you haven't found a decent doctor to help you. There really are some nice ones out there, but they might be difficult to find. I know some people who have gone through 13-20 urologists before finding one that was willing to work WITH them, listen to them, TALK to them even! Same thing with Naturopaths, NAET doctors, Acupuncturists, Physical Therapists, etc. There are good ones and bad ones in every field. If you have a good doctor, alternative or medical, consider yourself very fortunate. There are many IC patients who are not that lucky. And if you are among those less fortunate and haven't found a good urologist or you are in a country other than the U.S. where IC doctors are even more difficult to come by, then please know that you can still get better on your own. Please do not be without hope. I got better on my own and I know you can do it too.

As I always say, I was blessed in the end that I was never able to find a good urologist; that physically I was too sick, and financially I couldn't afford, to fly all over the country to see an "IC expert". At first I thought I was doomed. I thought there was no way I was ever going to get better if I didn't find a good doctor who knew all about IC. But in the end, not being able to find a doctor is what pushed me into treating myself and into finding answers that were not necessarily mainstream. It's like what Robert Frost said "To roads diverged in the woods. I took the one less traveled and it has made all the difference." Though I'm certainly not promoting going without a doctor if you have IC, I do believe that the fact that I didn't have one is how I ended up figuring this out. It's what made all the difference for me. And as much as this might freak some people out to hear, to be perfectly honest, it's how I got better. I got better because I took a different approach.

Now...in saying all that...I want to also say that I had a lot of trouble with alternatives as well. It's not like alternative doctors understand IC and know how to treat it either. However, I have to give them a lot of credit because at least they usually recognize the toxic body. At least they recognize right away that the IC patient is toxic and that they need to do some type of cleansing. They also usually recognize that the patient is sick all over the body, not just in the bladder. So I give them a lot of credit for that, but the problem is, they then usually recommend things that are much too harsh for someone who has IC. They often end up hurting the IC patient or causing them a setback, a flare, whatever you want to call it, because the natural products, herb, or supplements that they recommend are things that are often way too strong for someone with IC. I watch this happen all the time.

My first experience with an herbologist is the perfect example of what not to do. I went to see someone who was very knowledgeable about herbs and vitamins, but had never heard of IC. She didn't want to hear anything about it from me either. She wanted to muscle test me (kinesiology) and then tell me what to take; what she thought my body needed. She convinced me that she knew what she was doing and I proceeded to buy hundreds of dollars worth of vitamins, herbal supplements and Chinese herbs. I went home, did exactly what she told me to do and took a whole handful of these various supplements. I had a HUGE horrible reaction that I'll never forget the rest of my life. It was as if I had been poisoned. I got extremely sick and it took me days to recover. I might have needed all this nutrition, but my bladder and body could in no way handle them. And although this was a major lesson for me, I still had to learn it more than once before I finally "got it".

I know now that giving a toxic body tons of supplements is just asking for trouble. From my experience, it is NOT the right thing to do if you have IC. A person can become severely ill if they take too many nutrients at once when chronically toxic. The nutrients will cause a mad, uncontrolled release of toxins that the body is in no way prepared to release or handle. The result is, the person gets very sick. This is very often what happens to IC patients who go to herbologists, natural doctors of whatever type, or listen to their local health food store expert. Also, when the body is fighting chronic infection (which can also be the case with IC), it is using all of its energy for that purpose. Vitamin and mineral supplements can sometimes cause an increase or even a spread of yeast and viral infections. Often the supplements are too much for the digestive system and the body to handle, not to mention an IC bladder. **Just because a person has knowledge of vitamins, herbs, etc., does not mean they know how to prescribe them for an IC patient.** In fact, what I have learned is that the vast majority of them don't know how. The problem is, most of them will go ahead and tell you what to take anyway. Again, the responsibility is ours to know when to listen and when not to; to know when we have to do more research on our own first, or to know that we can't take anything strong or that we can't take 52 different things at once, etc. I've said this before in *To Wake In Tears* and I still feel this way. I don't believe there is such a thing as an IC expert. I believe that we have to be our own IC expert. We have to understand **our** IC enough so that we can prevent being hurt any further by either the medical or the naturals.

It took me a while to stop listening to what other people were telling me to take and to figure out what I should take on my own. Naturopaths, NAET doctors, chiropractors, osteopaths, homeopaths, herbologists, they are all wonderful resources for us. But just as I believe it's important to research into what your medical doctor or urologist is recommending you to do, I also believe it's just as important to do more research into what your alternative health care provider is recommending as well. I learned my lesson the hard way. I try to warn other IC patients about this, but most often they make the same mistake anyway. It's one of those things that we just seem to have to learn on our own. It's easy to fall into the trap of listening to someone who is a "professional" or an "expert". We want to believe them. We want them to have some answers for us. And although they all seem to tell us something different, when we are in the moment, talking to them and getting their advice, sometimes we decide to just go for it and "buy" whatever it is their selling. Whether it's an invasive procedure, a homeopathic remedy, a prescription medication, or an herbal combination, it seems we've all made this mistake. I know I've said this many times before, but we need to do as much research into the good and bad of each treatment and talk to other IC patients first before trying anything new. And after we do those two things, we need to listen to what our gut is telling us to do and follow that. And even when we follow our gut instincts, we often still need to proceed with extreme caution and go very slow (if possible) with the new treatment.

There is obviously good and bad in both the medical community and the "alternative" community. There are good and bad doctors, good and bad Naturopaths, Osteopaths, Acupuncturists, etc. There are good and bad treatments, good and bad ethics, and good and bad "medicines" on either side. Until that point somewhere in our future where alternative medicine and "modern" medicine join together for the welfare of the patient, we are stuck with the decision of going one way or the other. At the same time, there are many people who are combining both medical and alternative treatments on their own anyway. Actually, I'd have to say that the majority IC patients I talk to or "see" on line are doing just that. Although I completely understand why so many people are doing that (and I did the same exact thing initially), I do see problems with that approach. First and most obvious, problems can arise if the pharmaceutical medications happen to interact poorly with the natural products being taken. I can advise you to make sure to tell your doctor about all the natural products you're taking, but I know that many people don't or won't. They are either uncomfortable telling their doctor because their doctor will not "approve" or they don't tell them because they are aware that their doctor has little, if any, knowledge in that area. How will their doctor know if taking a particular herb or natural product will interfere with their medications when the doctor doesn't know anything about that herb or natural product? Herein lies one of the problems.

Another problem with combining medical and natural treatments can arise because often, in my opinion, what IC patients are taking pharmaceutical-wise is often working against what they are doing/taking natural-wise and vice versa. I believe this is one of the many possible reasons why alternative treatments haven't worked for some IC patients.

There are several reasons, I think, why alternative treatments haven't worked out so well for some IC patients and maybe why they haven't worked for you in the past if you've tried them. First, and possibly most often, the natural product chosen is too strong for someone as toxic and sensitive as an IC patient. I think this happens a lot. There are several herbs and natural products out there that are fantastic if you have a regular bladder infection, for example, but they are horrible for someone with IC. Cranberry juice is a great example of something natural that most people have heard of that is wonderful for regular bladder infections, but causes great pain for IC patients. Uva ursi is another great example. It's an herb that is wonderful for a normally healthy person with a regular bladder infection, but it can cause tremendous burning for someone with IC. Often what is recommended to an IC patient is appropriate for a regular bladder infection, but is completely inappropriate for an IC bladder.

Secondly, the natural product may be cleansing to the body and therefore causes a "reaction" that the patient may think means it is making them worse. And although the person may definitely feel worse and definitely has a worsening of symptoms, it may be a cleansing reaction and therefore it's really a "good" thing. In other words, it may be the "purpose" of the natural product to be producing these results (at least temporarily). But many people, after experiencing a worsening of symptoms, discontinue the natural product. They might even end up taking something synthetic to help with the cleansing symptoms. Usually they are unaware that the cleansing reaction is what is causing the increase in symptoms and therefore, understandably, the natural product is blamed. Colostrum is a good example. Some see it as an immune system booster (which it is) and don't necessarily realize that it's also a cleanser. Anything that causes cleansing can and often will increase IC symptoms. (This is why I talk about soothing more when cleansing.) But if you start taking Colostrum and don't realize that it's cleansing you (especially if you follow the directions on the side of the bottle, which in my opinion is way too strong a dose for an IC patient) and you don't soothe while you are taking it and drink plenty of water, it will most likely cause more burning and irritation as it pushes toxins from your body through the urine. This does not make Colostrum automatically "bad" for you and it also doesn't mean that it's not helping you either. It can be helping you and causing you an increase in symptoms at the same time. This can be the case with other herbs and natural products that cause an increase in IC symptoms as well, not just Colostrum.

Another reason why alternative treatments may not have worked for some people is because the natural product may not be "enough". Either not enough time is given or possibly it's just "not enough"; more needs to be done in order to get better. The natural product may be helping the person, but they just can't feel it yet or maybe it is helping, but it's not enough to get them better. In other words, some people expect an herb or natural product to produce results that they can feel right away (like they do with medications) and when they don't feel better right away, they think that the product is not working. I know IC patients who have been told to take Echinacea for example and so they take it for a while, they don't get better, and so they think Echinacea is no good; it didn't work. This happens with all kinds of alternative treatments, not just herbs. Also, the natural product might be theoretically great for IC or for the bladder, for example, but not necessarily great for the particular "phase" the individual is in with *their* IC. Or maybe it's something that is great for the bladder for normally healthy people, but not great for the bladder if you have IC, as I was saying earlier.

Something else that happens fairly often for IC patients is that they might be allergic to the natural herb/product that they tried. No matter how great an herb, how great a natural product, just like anything else, if the person is allergic to it, they will not have a good reaction and it certainly won't help them the way the herb/natural product is intended to. In fact, it will make them worse. Another reason might be that the person was taking too strong of a dose and so it affects them poorly. Where if they were to take a smaller dose of the same thing, it might not. In fact, a smaller dose of that same herb/natural product that was previously causing problems just might turn out to be VERY beneficial. I believe that due to our extreme toxicity and sensitivity, often it is a lower dose that is necessary for us to be able to tolerate much of anything. (Naturally, this is especially so for those with severe IC.)

And lastly, something that I feel happens very frequently, the natural product may be inhibited by the synthetic/chemical medications that are being taken at the same time. In other words, if someone is taking several medications or even one synthetic medication and is also taking some natural things, often they will not be getting the same benefits from the natural things that a person taking no medications would be getting. For example, many IC patients who have read *To Wake In Tears* decided to try drinking marshmallow root tea. At the same time, they naturally continued on with their other medications. Whether it be Elmiron, anti-depressants such as Elavil or Doxepin, anti-histamines, anti-inflammatories, pain medications, etc., many who were or are trying marshmallow root tea to soothe their bladder are also taking some combination of these various synthetic medications. They then write or call me and ask why they're not better yet. Remember, marshmallow root is a purifier. And while it soothes and nourishes the bladder lining, it is also gently flushing the body of toxins. The more chemicals being added to the body (whether through medications or other sources), the more work the body has to do to flush the chemicals/toxins out. The more toxic the urine, the more irritation there will be to the bladder, again, the harder the job for the marshmallow root.

Also, you can't just drink marshmallow root tea and expect that to be enough. I hear from so many people who tell me they're drinking marshmallow root tea and they want to know why they aren't better yet. Yes, marshmallow root is going to help your bladder lining to heal, but if you're taking all kinds of synthetic medications and/or still have other sources of toxins in place, it will not be enough. It will not be nearly enough. If your sources of toxins remain in place, it will not be enough to drink marshmallow root tea to get you better. Your body will continually have to process those toxins and will therefore continue to cause irritation to your bladder and to the rest of you.

I know a lot of people out there are drinking marshmallow root tea and taking Elmiron. So many have written me with this question that I wanted to make sure and address it in this book. Although I understand the logic of why people are doing this, I have to be honest and say that I don't think it's a good idea for a couple of reasons. First of all, as I said, marshmallow root is a purifier. It is gently cleansing the body of impurities and soothing the tissues at the same time. When you take a purifier with a chemical, synthetic medication, it may 1) reduce the effects of the medication and 2) it will also cause the marshmallow root to be less effective. So even though it seems like you are doubling up on your "soothers" to the bladder, in reality, you may be making them both work less effectively. Personally, I would choose one or the other and not take them together. Naturally, I would start off with marshmallow root first because to me, it is much less of a risk. Elmiron is still relatively new to the market and though there are several known short-term side effects (e.g., possible hair loss, stomach upset, headaches), it hasn't been long enough yet to know if there are any long-term side effects. At $2.00 a bag for a 4-6 month supply, not to mention that it is natural, non-toxic, and without side effects (for those not allergic of course), I feel marshmallow root is a much safer choice. Another plus is that marshmallow root is not hard on the kidneys and liver, quite the contrary actually. To me, there are so many more advantages to marshmallow root, but as I always say, do what you feel most comfortable with.

Many have written me about taking aloe vera and marshmallow root together. There is no conflict there if you ask me. Both are natural purifiers and healers that soothe the tissues. It is my belief that aloe vera is better for the intestines, where marshmallow root tea is better for the bladder, but there are a lot of people who find aloe vera helpful for their bladder. Even comfrey leaf and marshmallow root together are fine. All of them are natural purifiers and soothers and will not be "fighting" each other.

Some wonder whether the Elmiron is coating the bladder and therefore not allowing the marshmallow root to get into the tissues to help them heal. I would have to agree. If the Elmiron is effectively coating the bladder lining, I'm not sure how well the marshmallow root would be able to be absorbed. Again, I'd have to say that I wouldn't recommend taking them together. At the same time, I don't think it's going to out and out hurt you either. I believe it will just cause both to be less effective.

Maybe you have tried alternative treatments in the past and they not only didn't help you, but they might have even made you worse. Maybe one or more of the above reasons contributed to why. Maybe you are someone who is combining both alternative and medical treatments and you're not sure what is helping and what is hurting. Hopefully some of the warnings in this section will help you to be able to determine why you're not getting better yet or maybe why you've had a setback.

I think more and more people are learning or realizing that just because something is natural does not mean that it's safe; it does not mean that it can't hurt you. You can be allergic to natural herbs and organic foods, the same way that you can be allergic to medications and synthetic products. Our bodies all have different sensitivities. Only we can know our bodies well enough and keep track of all these sensitivities. (By the way, NAET is great for this.)

It is my opinion that failing to remove the sources of poison/toxins to your body will prevent you from getting well. It's another reason why alternative treatments may not have worked for some people. You can cleanse and get rid of candida, for example, and stick to the anti-candida diet religiously, but if you don't remove the sources, the candida will come right back. I've seen this happen so many times, not only with IC patients, but other people who have candida as well. I believe it's one of the reasons why systemic candida is so difficult for some people to get over. You can take Diflucan over and over, do a whole big natural anti-candida program, even stick to the anti-candida diet religiously, and still the yeast will come right back. This is what happened to me as well. But once I removed the sources of poison to my body, I have had no problems with the candida returning. Take the toxic environment away and they'll have no place to play. The same goes with bacteria thriving in a toxic environment. Until I removed the sources of toxins, I got infections of all kinds all the time. I caught every little thing that was going around (and even some things that weren't). I could have continued to boost my immune system all the time and continued to cleanse, but if I hadn't removed the sources, my immune system would be continually overworked and compromised. The main sources I'm talking about here are mercury and cigarettes (for me). Also, if I didn't replace the vitamins and minerals that I was lacking, I could not have gotten all the way better. I could have gotten to a certain point, which I did. But I could not have returned to a state of normal health without re-balancing my body and rebuilding it with nutrition. Once I got to that point and figured out what I was lacking in terms of vitamins and minerals, then I was able to move on and get the rest of the way better. (See Section 5 for more information about vitamins and minerals.)

The following are some things that not only I ran into, but also what many other IC patients have run into. It's funny how so many of us made the same mistakes. Well okay, it's not funny. But maybe you can learn from our mistakes and avoid them. If you have fairly mild IC, some of these warnings may not totally apply to you. You probably won't be AS sensitive as someone who has moderate to severe IC. So keep in mind that you may be able to experiment a little more with things that someone with a more severe case of IC could not. As I always say, listen to your body, look to your own situation, and listen to your own judgment of what to do. Don't just go by what I say or what any one person tells you. I think also that I may be overly cautious because my IC was so severe and my bladder and body were so insanely sensitive because of it. At the same time, I have seen others in the same exact boat, experiencing the same exact things and making the same exact mistakes I made. So that's why I felt it was very important to share these warnings with you.

Be careful of ANYTHING that is strong. Any natural product or medication that is considered strong for "normal" people is something I would be *extremely* careful of if you have IC. The more severe your IC, the more sensitive you probably are and the more careful you will need to be. Speaking of avoiding things that are too strong....

Be careful of homeopathic remedies and Chinese herbs in general because both are often very strong. Homeopathy and Chinese herbs are really terrific for certain things, but IC, in my opinion, is not one of them. I know countless IC patients, myself included, who have had terrible reactions from homeopathic remedies. The basis of homeopathy is that like cures like. Give the body a little of what it's fighting and it'll boost the immune system into fighting it harder. This is also the basis of allergy shots, flu shots, and vaccinations, by the way. They were born out of homeopathy, which was extremely popular before "modern" medicine came along. All of these are things that personally I would avoid having IC. I don't believe we are strong enough or well enough to handle these things. At the same time, you might be able to. We are all different. And if you are someone that benefits from a flu shot or didn't have trouble with a homeopathic remedy, then I think that's great. But in my opinion, most IC patients will probably not be able to.

Be careful of following directions on the side of the bottle when it comes to herbs and supplements. Keep in mind that those directions are often for 150 lbs., normally healthy adults. Those dosages are probably going to be way too strong for an IC patient. Also remember that when it comes to herbs and supplements, we will not all be the same in terms of what is the correct dosage. It will depend on several factors, a couple of them being your body weight and how much your bladder and body can tolerate. Start out with the smallest dosage you possibly can. Open the capsule, crunch up the pill (but first make sure it's not the time release kind), and at the most, take only one pill or one capsule the first time you try it.

Be careful of running into an alternative doctor or herbologist who wants to sell you all kinds of supplements or tells you that they need to detoxify you. It has been my experience that natural or alternative type doctors, though AT LEAST they recognize a toxic body, don't understand the massive sensitivity of an IC patient and will try to get you to do things that are going to end up hurting you. Please listen to their advice and then go home and do some research first. As I've said before, there is nothing wrong with doing some research on your own just to make sure. You will save yourself a lot of money and possible setbacks by taking this approach. Some examples of things they may want you to try but that I believe will probably be too strong include the following: homeopathic remedies, cleansing herbal combinations, chelation therapy, colonics, hydrogen peroxide IV treatments, liver or lymphatic cleanses, desensitization drops, hydrochloric acid, and various nutritional supplements. Naturally this is not to say that there is anything "wrong" with any of these therapies or things, just that in my opinion many IC patients probably won't be able to handle them.

Be careful of running into someone at the health food store that thinks they know what you should take and how you should take it. A person at a health food store, no matter how much knowledge they have about herbs and vitamins, will NOT understand IC and will most likely lead you to buying products that are going to bother you and maybe even hurt you. They will not understand how sensitive you are or how toxic. They will recommend things that are good for the bladder, but not necessarily for an IC bladder. Again, Uva Ursi is a good example. It's a great herb for the urinary tract and for regular cystitis, but for most IC patients it's going to be way too strong and can cause a lot of pain. There are many herbs and natural products that might be good for the bladder in a normally healthy person, but they are not going to be appropriate for IC. If you get advice from someone at the health food store, just like if you get advice from an alternative type doctor, do yourself a big favor. Don't buy the stuff on the spot. Instead, go home and research into it further. Again, don't just take one person's advice, mine included.

Be careful of running into a natural dentist who tries to convince you that you need to spend thousands of dollars and go through this whole huge procedure to have your fillings replaced. Many people, looking to have their mercury fillings replaced, end up going to a natural dentist who not only charges a small fortune (e.g., 4-5 thousand dollars), but scares the person half to death with their description of how the mercury must be removed carefully with these expensive procedures and how the patient will need to do an extensive de-toxing program in order to remove the mercury from the tissues of the body. But to go to this extreme and to charge that kind of money is not really necessary if you ask me. Now it is true that we need to be careful when removing the fillings because it is, after all, a poison. Even regular ADA dentists are told to dispose of the removed fillings as toxic waste, because that's what it is. (Scary to think that it's considered toxic waste the minute it is removed from our mouths, but it's supposed to be non-toxic and harmless to us when it was is in our mouth two minutes before...?) And the de-tox programs, which typically contain high doses of vitamin C and all kinds of other supplements, will just about kill most IC patients. It's just way too strong, in my opinion. At the same time, it IS true that we need to cleanse the mercury from our bodies. It's not enough to just remove the fillings. The body has been exposed to the poison from the fillings for a long time and almost always there is some that has been stored in the body. And it is also true that we have to be careful when having the fillings removed. We should try not to breathe in the mercury vapors (breathe through your nose) and try not to swallow any of the pieces of the filling that are being drilled out.

Many people ask me about this and how I did it. I had my fillings replaced by my regular ADA dentist. To this day he has no idea that I thought my fillings had anything to do with my health. We never discussed it. I went in and told him that my doctor tested me and found me to be allergic to mercury and therefore recommended that I have my fillings replaced. He said, "Okay we can do that". He was wonderful about it and very patient with me as I took several bathroom breaks during appointments (obviously he knew all about me having IC and needing to take breaks). I was also very fortunate that it ended up being covered by my insurance. I think maybe it was covered because I had told my dentist that I was allergic to mercury. (By the way, my NAET doctor is the one who tested me, but it was really me who wanted to have my fillings replaced. Although I could have easily proven it to be the case, neither my dentist nor my insurance company requested proof that I was allergic to mercury.)

ADA dentists are not allowed to say anything bad about mercury fillings. They can loose their license if they do. Especially if they tell you that your fillings have anything at all to do with your health problems. I know a lot of people who have run into the problem that their normal ADA dentist refuses to remove their fillings. It has been my experience that if you go in there and tell your dentist that you want to have your fillings replaced because you think that they are "causing" your health problems (or has anything at all to do with your health) that many ADA dentists will then refuse to remove them. I think they are worried 1) about liability if you don't get better after they remove them, and 2) they are taught that mercury amalgam fillings are safe and that the mercury does not leak out. If you want your regular dentist to replace your fillings, I would just tell them something similar to what I told mine and not mention, or even hint at, that you think your fillings are causing you health problems. Because I had told my dentist that I was allergic to mercury, he understood my concern over having any of the filling fragments go down my throat accidentally so he placed an extra cotton gauze pad in my mouth to block that from happening. I also breathed through my nose while he was drilling so as not to breathe in as much of the mercury vapors.

As I mentioned in *To Wake In Tears*, I used Colostrum to gently cleanse the mercury from my body throughout the time that I was having my fillings replaced and also for a few months after. It has been over a year and a half since I had my last filling replaced and I am still getting better all the time. It takes time for all the poison to work its way out of the gums and tissues. Don't expect to be better in 5 minutes after having your fillings replaced. It will more than likely take some time. If you have a lot of fillings and you are in the middle of having them replaced, you might even feel worse temporarily until you finish having them all removed. That's what happened to me. The teeth I still had fillings in were bothering me even more than they did before I started having them replaced. And some of them that I had replaced were pretty sensitive. It took some time before that sensitivity went away. It takes time for the poison to work its way out through the gums and for the nerves in the teeth to heal. Though I could tell a huge difference right away, probably because I had so many fillings (13), I knew it was going to take some time for all that poison to clear out of my system. And it has. But I have continued to get better and better since then with no setbacks and no new symptoms. I guess because of the IC and having to go slow with de-toxing, it is taking me longer to cleanse out the mercury than it would have for someone who doesn't have IC and did one of the more aggressive de-toxing programs with a natural dentist.

By the way, if you feel more comfortable going to a natural dentist to have this done, then by all means, do so. I'm sure it is probably a safer way to go. Like I always say, don't do what I did just because it's what I did. Do what makes you feel the most comfortable.

Be careful of taking a large combination of things, even if they are all natural things, but especially be careful of taking a combination of natural and synthetic/chemical medications. If you take too many different things at the same time, not only is it confusing to know what is helping you, but it can also be very hard on your body. You can be taking 7-10 different natural products and not be feeling any better and the reason might be because you are taking 7-10 different natural products. In my opinion, you might be better off cutting back and keeping it simple. One of the things that I did that I feel helped me a lot in getting better was to not overdo anything. I didn't take a whole bunch of stuff at one time. Keeping it simple made it easier to know what was going on and most importantly made it easier on my body as well.

Be careful when taking pharmaceutical medications. Unfortunately FDA approval and rigorous testing does not guarantee that a person can't have a negative reaction to a medication. Personally, I have taken prescribed medications from my doctor that I had very horrible reactions to and these medications were/are FDA approved. I'm sure this has happened to many people, but especially IC patients because we are typically extra sensitive. In reality, there is always the risk that the treatment you try can make you worse. Sadly, it's rare that you hear about that risk before the treatment. I mean, a doctor will most likely say to you, "Okay, let's go with the DMSO first", for example. "It might help and it might not, but we'll try it first." He never says, "Oh and by the way, not only is there a chance it won't help you, but there is also the risk that it can make you worse". It's that way for all bladder instillations, not just DMSO. It's that way for hydrodistentions and even for something like Elmiron too. I realize there are some people that find relief through those things, but there are also some people who actually get much worse from them. There are people who have had these procedures or who have taken these medications that never seem to get better after doing them. I don't think it's right that often we are not told of the risk that we can get worse. I've certainly never read about that risk in any of the IC literature. But I have heard doctors and pharmacists deny that it's possible though. They claim that these treatments and medications could not be to blame. But if you talk to IC patients who have lived through the experience, they will tell you MUCH differently. This is, again, why it's SO important to talk to other IC patients prior to going through any treatment. The same goes for alternative treatments. There are some alternative treatments that can also make you worse too; it's not just the medical ones.

Be careful of taking multiple antibiotics or multiple cleansers. I just spoke with an IC patient this afternoon that was taking antibiotics for a regular UTI, Echinacea/goldenseal, olive leaf extract, and garlic. At the same time, she was taking a colon cleanse to fight yeast (which she felt she got from taking so many antibiotics in the past). She was presently taking 4 antibiotics at the same time, a synthetic antibiotic and three natural ones. Not only is it not really necessary, it can be very hard on the body to take multiple antibiotics and/or multiple cleansing products. It can make you feel much worse, put you more out of balance, and also put too much of a strain on your body making it more difficult to heal. Again, more is not always better.

Remember, if you're taking herbs and natural products, that it's a good idea to take breaks sometimes. It is that way for everyone, not just IC patients. But especially for us because we can more easily develop a sensitivity or resistance to something. Many of you will know what I am talking about when I say that IC patients can take a certain medication for a period of time and do really well with it...and then it will stop working...or worse yet...it will actually start to cause more problems. This happens a lot. We develop a resistance to or sensitivity to that which was previously helping us. Taking breaks from things that are helping us will help prevent this from happening.

Section 4

Herbs and IC

Obviously I am not an herbologist. However, I can share with you what I have learned from researching on my own, talking to herbologists, and personally using the following herbs while I was healing from IC. As always, I would recommend looking to several sources for information on herbs, natural products, and even pharmaceutical medications.

Herbs are not like medications in that they are not to cover symptoms, but rather to help the body to heal. So it can, and usually does, take longer to feel relief when using herbs. At the same time, there are some herbs that do provide "immediate" results. With herbs, there is much less chance of causing chemical toxicity within the body. To me, this is a very important fact for IC patients who, in my opinion, already have chemical toxicity within the body to begin with.

As you probably know, we can be allergic to any herb or any synthetic medication. So we have to be careful of both. I would always **start very slowly** with each new herb (or really anything) I ever tried. This would minimize the chance of having a bad reaction. If I were to drink a few sips of herbal tea and I turned out to be allergic to that herb (or if it bothered my bladder), obviously I would not have to go through as horrible of a reaction as I would have had I drank a full cup. Something else I think was really important was that I would only **try one thing at a time**. It really made a big difference in being able to tell whether the new thing I tried was hurting or helping.

87

I think **single herbs are best** for IC patients. Once you get into herbal combinations, whether in capsules, tinctures, or teabags, it increases the odds that you won't be able to tolerate them. By taking one herb at a time, there is more likelihood that you will find herbs that you can tolerate.

Herbs can be taken (and used) in many forms. They can be taken in capsules, tinctures, and teas. They can be used in a bath or in a poultice. How you take the herb is decided based on what you are trying to accomplish. For example, herbal tinctures are a concentrated liquid form of the herb that you normally take under your tongue. Some people put the drops in water or use it to make tea, but most often it is taken under the tongue. Herbs taken in a tincture are absorbed quickly and go directly into the blood (when taken under the tongue). Herbs taken in capsule form are swallowed, dissolved in the stomach and are best absorbed throughout the digestives system. And herbs taken in a tea form are best absorbed throughout all the tissues.

I think **using herbs in tea form for IC patients has many advantages**. For one thing, you can make the tea as weak as you want and only take a few sips at a time. Many of us are very sensitive and where an entire capsule of an herb might be hard on us, taking a few sips of the herb in a tea can be very helpful and much easier to handle. Taking the slow approach and taking small doses made a huge difference for me. I found that erring on the side of caution and going slow was much easier than dealing with a setback or a strong allergic reaction. Other reasons that I think using herbs in tea form is great for IC patients are that 1) we don't have to digest the gelatin capsules that herbs often come in which can aggravate the stomach and intestines for some IC patients, 2) we can buy the herbs in bulk form (or loose form) which is very inexpensive and we can see exactly what we're getting, 3) we can take a very low dose of the herb which might be all that we can handle, and 4) we can get nutrition (vitamins and minerals) from herb tea that is much easier for our body to absorb and easier to tolerate bladder-wise.

Marshmallow Root (the herb, the tincture, and the capsules)
What does it do? Marshmallow root has been called the "aloe vera for internal organs". It is very soothing and healing to all mucous membranes due to its high mucilage content. Made into a tea, marshmallow root is excellent for soothing and nourishing the lining of the bladder, kidneys, and entire urinary tract. Marshmallow root is a purifier and helps gently (very gently) cleanse the body of impurities and toxins and soothes the tissues at the same time. According to Michael Moore, author of "Herbs for the Urinary Tract", marshmallow root is "...probably the single most useful herb...for soothing the bladder, ureters, and urethra membranes after recuperating from an infection, stone episode or a bout of interstitial cystitis. It also acts as an immunostimulant and often seems to improve the membrane health as well."[1]

Why is it good for IC patients? In my opinion, there are several reasons why marshmallow root is a great herb for many IC patients. Marshmallow root tea is very soothing to an inflamed and/or bleeding IC bladder. It not only acts as an anti-inflammatory, it will actually help nourish the tissues to help them heal. It will help with bladder spasms, bladder pain, inability to initiate the urine stream, and will help increase the flow of urine. In other words, there will be more force behind the urine stream. Most important is the soothing support that marshmallow root will provide an IC bladder (kidneys, urethra and entire urinary tract). The capsules are great for the intestines, the glycerin based (non-alcohol) tincture is great for pain in the kidneys and bladder, and the tea is great for all of the above and especially for the helping to heal and soothe the bladder lining. Marshmallow root is also alkalizing to the body and to the urine, which is extremely helpful to IC patients who often have a very acidic body.

As I mentioned in *To Wake In Tears*, I found marshmallow root to be extremely helpful in helping my bladder lining to heal. Since then, many people have written or called me with similar questions regarding marshmallow root which I wanted to make sure to address in this book.

First let me say that marshmallow root, like any other herb, medication, or treatment, is not an answer for everyone. But if you can tolerate it (and from what I've seen, a large percentage of IC patients can), it can be very helpful in healing and soothing your bladder, kidneys, and urinary tract. But of course there will be people who are allergic to marshmallow root, just like anything else. It doesn't matter that marshmallow root is soothing. Just like aloe vera. They are both soothing type things, but if you are allergic to them, then they aren't going to help you. (Actually they will cause you more trouble, which is usually how you end up figuring it out.) One way to find out if marshmallow root is going to bother you without ingesting any is to put a very small amount on your tongue. If you don't get any reaction (like nausea for example), you have a better chance of being okay with it. Even still I would start with only a couple sips the first time you try it. You should be able to tell from a fairly small amount whether it bothers you or not. The first time you try it, I would advise you to NOT drink a whole or even a half of a cup. I would advise the same when trying any new herb.

Marshmallow root is one of the most soothing and mellow herbs out there. It's one of the very few herbs considered safe for babies and pregnant women (how many things can we say that about?) It's soothing because of its high mucilage content. It should NOT cause burning. It should ease burning and there should be no side effects unless you are allergic to it. Please also keep in mind that marshmallow root is a purifier. It is helping to gently flush your system of toxins and junk. This is really a good thing, but I think that many people make the tea fairly strong and then they feel the flush as an increase in burning. If you have Vulvodynia or you're very toxic, even something as mild and gentle as marshmallow root, due to the "flush", can cause an increase in burning when you first start to use it. If that has happened to you, you might want to try to make the tea weaker. It does NOT have to be strong for it to work and you don't have to drink a ton of it either. You don't even have to be ultra religious about how much or when you drink it. You can drink marshmallow root tea with food, without food, or at any time of day. Small amounts WILL help and you will be less likely to feel the "flush" of toxins. However, I would recommend being near a bathroom when you drink it. Marshmallow root tea does have mild diuretic properties. Like any other herb tea, it will cause your frequency to increase temporarily until it passes through you. It's just like if you drank regular iced tea, soda, or a couple of beers. You go to the bathroom more often until it passes through you. This is the only "symptom" that should be noticed when drinking marshmallow root tea. And for some people who experience bladder spasms and "pee freeze" this "symptom" will bring much needed relief. For me, it was one of the many benefits of drinking marshmallow root tea. It should help with those who have trouble emptying their bladder all the way. At least, it helped me with that symptom.

How to use it? I used to use the glycerin based (non-alcohol) tincture for severe pain in my bladder and/or kidneys. I would put a few drops of the tincture under the tongue during extra painful times, let it sit for a second or two, and then follow with some water. I used to take the capsules for my intestines. The capsules are soothing to the tissues of the stomach and intestines, just as the tea is to the bladder. If you take the capsules for your bladder, you will most likely not feel or get the same effect as you would if you drink the tea. As you probably already know, I drank marshmallow root tea the most often and I did so to help soothe and heal my bladder and kidneys.

Many people call or write asking me if it's okay to use the capsules to make tea because they can't find a place to get the actual root in bulk form. It is my opinion that the tea (made from the root or even the leaf) is the ideal. But if you already bought the capsules because you couldn't find the root and you want to make tea from the capsule, then that will be okay. It's definitely better than nothing. But making it from the root (or even the leaf) is the best in my opinion. Others have asked me if it's okay to just swallow the capsules because they don't want to bother with making the tea or they don't like the taste or whatever. There is nothing wrong with taking the capsules. I mean...they will benefit your bladder some. But just remember, capsules taken (not made into tea, but swallowed whole) are best absorbed in the stomach and digestive system. The marshmallow root capsules will therefore be more beneficial to your intestines than they will be to your bladder. The tea is best absorbed throughout all the tissues. (This is not just marshmallow root, but with any herb you're taking in tea or capsule form.) Naturally some people are going to do better with capsules than with teas, again because we are all different. BUT for the most part, it is my opinion/experience that drinking the tea made from the actual root is the best thing for the bladder (and kidneys.)

If you're interested and because so many people ask me all the time, here is one place that you can buy the root (they sell internationally) – Hannah Kroeger 1-303-443-0755 (www.hannahsherbshop.com). It's 90 cents for one ounce, so you can spend less than $1.00 to try marshmallow root if you're interested in trying it. Please note that I have no association whatsoever with this company. I've just used their stuff and found them reputable. I included this especially for those who don't have access to a computer, because sometimes marshmallow root is difficult to find locally.

If you know you're not allergic to marshmallow root (maybe you've been tested with NAET for it for example), but it still seems to cause you some burning and/or an increase in discharge and therefore an increase in Vulvodynia symptoms, there are a couple things you can do. You can take one eyedropper full of marshmallow root tea and put it in a glass of water. Drink a few sips of that the first time and then slowly increase until you can handle drinking a whole glass of water with one eyedropper full of tea in it. You can work your way up slowly to eventually adding 2-3 eyedroppers of tea to a glass of water until you can drink the weak tea on its own. Or obviously, you can choose another herb or natural product to help soothe your bladder. But if you know you're not allergic to it and would like to use it, this very slow process has helped several people I know.

How to make the tea…Some people have heard from health food store clerks or have read in herb books that marshmallow root tea should be made from a cold infusion; that the mucilage is greater when made cold versus hot. This may be true, but I never made it cold once and it worked great for me. You can make it any way you want (obviously) but making it hot will not destroy the mucilage, of this you can be sure. In fact, I would recommend making it weaker versus stronger anyway. I know some people steep it or boil it for 10-15 minutes. Personally, I think that's too long and makes the tea very strong. But if you can handle it that way, that's great. Roughly one tablespoon of the root to approximately 7 cups of water in a drip coffeemaker is the way I used to make it. If you're making it one cup at a time, just use a half teaspoon (it doesn't have to be exact) of the root in a tea ball and then dunk it a few times into a cup of hot water and there you have it. You don't have to let the tea ball sit steeping in the water. The tea should look a very light pale yellow color and it shouldn't taste like much of anything. If it tastes icky, it's too strong; too strong in my opinion of course. Once brewed, I used to pour the tea over a couple of ice cubes to cool it down and weaken it further. (Drinking anything too hot or too cold will "shock" or stress our system. This is true for anyone. And with IC, being so sensitive to EVERYTHING, I thought it best to drink my herb teas warm versus piping hot. Naturally this was just the way I did it. Obviously, you should do whatever you're most comfortable with.) If you can only find the capsules and have to use those to make a tea, then I would just dump one capsule into a mug of hot water or a half a capsule into a smaller cup of hot water and stir. If you can only find marshmallow leaf, that will also work okay.

How much to drink… As I said, personally, I would start out with a few sips the first time. But I think that's important to do when trying any herb for the first time. As long as you feel nothing, which is what you should feel after a few sips of marshmallow root tea, then I would increase it to a half cup. Once you know that a half of a cup doesn't bother you, you can work your way up to a full cup and then 2-3 cups a day. The way I did it varied. Some days I drank 3-5 cups, some days 1-2. It depended on how I felt. You can't really overdo it when it comes to marshmallow root in terms of overdosing on it or anything, but if you drink a ton of it then there is a chance that it might cause diarrhea. And really, you don't want to overdo anything. Moderation, or erring on the side of less, is often the better move when you have IC. You would think logically that if something is good for you, then more is better. But with IC, this is not necessarily the case.

Contains: Marshmallow root is high in Vitamin A, magnesium, iron, and selenium. It is rich in protein and calcium and has moderate amounts of vitamin C, phosphorus, potassium, and manganese. It also contains small amounts of niacin, B1, B2, silicon, and zinc.[2]

Cautions: I could not find any warnings about marshmallow root in any of my herb books.

Comfrey Leaf (the herb)
What does it do? Due to its high mucilage content, Comfrey is very moistening and lubricating to all mucous membranes. Some say Comfrey has the highest percentage of mucilage of any herb. It has been used for centuries internally to help heal ulcers and externally to heal wounds and even broken bones. It is also very nourishing and soothing to the tissues of the stomach, intestines, lungs, kidneys, and bladder. Comfrey helps promote tissue growth in the body.[3] It is soothing and healing to ulcers and inflammation. Comfrey also absorbs toxins from the intestines and helps regulate intestinal flora.[4] Comfrey leaves are anti-inflammatory.

Why is it good for IC patients? The high mucilage content of comfrey, its anti-inflammatory action, the fact that it is nutritive and healing to the tissues, as well as its ability to gently cleanse the body are all excellent reasons why it might benefit some IC patients. Not only will comfrey help heal the bladder lining; it will also help absorb toxins from the intestines. Comfrey helps promote tissue growth in the body and is soothing and nourishing to mucous membranes. Although I believe it can be a great herb for some IC patients, comfrey does gently cleanse the liver and therefore it may be strong for some IC patients who are still very toxic. You don't want to overdo it with the comfrey, but it can be an excellent addition to your healing plan if used properly. Drinking comfrey leaf tea is also an excellent source of B-complex vitamins for IC patients because it is easily absorbed by the body and is much easier to tolerate bladder-wise because of its soothing mucilage quality.

How to use it? I used comfrey leaf in a tea. I found it very helpful in terms of helping my bladder lining to heal, but I only used it few times a week. Initially, I drank it alone to make sure I wasn't allergic/sensitive to it. Once I knew it didn't bother me, I added it to my marshmallow root tea a few times a week. Just because many people ask me, I used about a level teaspoon of the comfrey leaf, along with my usual tablespoon of marshmallow root, and then added approximately 7-8 cups of water to my drip coffeemaker. I used comfrey most often in my healing baths where I would throw a teaspoon or two into a tea ball and then throw it into the tub.

Contains: Comfrey is rich in Vitamin A, Vitamin C, and trace minerals. It is high in protein, calcium, potassium, phosphorus, and iron. Comfrey contains moderate amounts of magnesium, sulphur, and zinc, as well as small amounts of selenium. Along with 18 amino acids, comfrey also contains some B-complex vitamins, including B12, which is usually only found in animal protein.[5]

Cautions: Avoid if pregnant, nursing, or if you have liver disease. Also, comfrey is not for prolonged use in children.[6] Some sources warn against using comfrey internally and others rave about comfrey's benefits for internal use. (This is a good example of why it's important to check with several sources before using an herb.) The warnings are usually in reference to the liver because comfrey cleanses a toxic liver. The more toxic your liver, the slower you might want to go with comfrey. This is why comfrey root is no longer sold individually, though it is still added to herbal combinations. The leaf is not as strong as the root and that's why the leaf is still available for use on it's own. Due to the warnings, I was careful not to use comfrey every day and I would certainly not advise overdoing it by drinking several cups a day or anything. But using comfrey in moderation, in my opinion, can be very helpful in healing and soothing the bladder.

Parsley (the herb)

What does it do? "A study published in the Journal of Allergy and Clinical Immunology shows parsley inhibits the secretion of histamine, a chemical the body produces that triggers allergy symptoms."[7] Parsley is good for kidney inflammation, bladder inflammation and infection, and is helpful when there is urine retention due to its gentle diuretic properties. It is often used for fluid retention and edema. Parsley is healing to the urinary tract and is said to strengthen the kidneys and the uterus.[8] Parsley provides a toxic kidney with essential nutrients that aid in its cleansing. It is also nourishing for the stomach and helps indigestion and assimilation.[9] Parsley is also somewhat stimulating to the immune system. It helps to eliminate excess mucous and therefore acts as a decongestant.[10]

Why is it good for IC patients? Parsley tea can be a helpful gentle diuretic for IC patients who have trouble initiating the stream and/or emptying their bladder fully. Parsley, either eaten fresh or made into a tea, can be helpful to IC patients due to its antihistamine action (many IC patients have mast cells or histamines in their bladder), and it's ability to soothe the kidneys and bladder. Parsley will also provide nutritional support for the kidneys and urinary system. However, if you have Vulvodynia symptoms with your IC, then you might not want to use parsley because it is high in oxalates (which are said to aggravate Vulvodynia in some people). Otherwise, if an IC patient can tolerate it, I think parsley is an excellent food/herb for IC. I was able to add fresh parsley to my diet by adding it to my salads and I also used dried parsley sometimes in my marshmallow root tea. I also used parsley in my healing baths to help with bloating and edema.

How to use it? Parsley can be used in a tea as a gentle diuretic and to help soothe the kidneys and bladder. You can add a little to your marshmallow root tea or you can eat fresh raw parsley. You can also use it in the bath for edema and bloating. Just throw a pinch or two of dried parsley (just like you'd find at the grocery store) into a tea ball with whatever other herbs you are adding to your bath.

Contains: Parsley is rich in vitamin A, C, iron, chlorophyll, potassium, and sodium. It is high in calcium, phosphorus, sulphur, and the B-complex vitamins. Parsley also contains small amounts of selenium, zinc, and other trace minerals.[11]

Cautions: I couldn't find any cautions regarding parsley.

Raspberry Leaf (the herb)
What does it do? Raspberry Leaf supports and strengthens the walls of the uterus and all of the female reproductive organs. It is a uterine relaxant that also relaxes intestinal spasms. It is soothing to the mucous membranes and especially to the kidneys. It is good for bowel problems, mouth sores, sore throats, ulcers, and problems of the urinary tract.[12] Raspberry leaf helps dispel toxins from the body, helps eliminate mucous from the system, aids digestion and provides iron and calcium to the body.[13] Some people say that it very gently helps cleanse and purify the blood.

Why is it good for IC patients? Mellow and soothing to the bladder, raspberry leaf can be very beneficial to an IC patient. Raspberry leaf helps to calm the intestinal spasms of IBS. It is also very helpful to drink before and during your menstrual cycle to help support your female organs and to help ease cramps.

How to use it? Personally, I would recommend using raspberry leaf in a tea, rather than the capsule or tincture. You can make it plain by using a teaspoon to a tablespoon of the herb to 5-6 cups of water. (Adjust the amounts based on how strong you would like to make it. Keep in mind that I made all of my herb teas weak.) The way I used raspberry leaf the most was to make marshmallow root tea with one tablespoon of the root, a teaspoon of catnip and a teaspoon of raspberry leaf thrown into the gold filter of my drip coffeemaker and then added to 8-9 cups of water. This is the tea mixture I drank around my menstrual cycle for cramps and also for the intestinal spasms of IBS. It provides immediate relief and it doesn't taste half bad.

Contains: Raspberry leaf is rich in manganese, iron, and niacin. It is high in calcium, magnesium, selenium, vitamin A and vitamin C. It also contains moderate amounts of phosphorus, potassium, and B-complex vitamins, along with trace amounts of sodium, silicon, and zinc.[14]

Cautions: I couldn't find any cautions for raspberry leaf.

Cat's Claw (the capsules or the herb)
What does it do? Cat's Claw (also called Una de Gato) is great for boosting the immune system and supporting the intestines. It supports the intestinal tract by helping to cleanse it and also by soothing it. It is also said to provide anti-inflammatory support for the whole body. South American herbologists have used this herb for centuries to treat ulcers, digestive problems, arthritis, and other inflammatory ailments.

Why is it good for IC patients? Because Cat's Claw is a gentle cleanser of the colon and is great for boosting the immune system, I think it's a good herb for IC patients to try. I used it mostly to boost my immune system and for me it wasn't too hard on the bladder. But, as we all know, we are all different. So go very slow the first time you try it to make sure it doesn't bother you.

How to use it? Because I had heard that the tea doesn't taste too good and also since I was taking it for my intestines and immune system, I decided to take it in capsule form. Cat's Claw can be hard on the stomach for some people, especially if taken everyday. If I would have taken it every day, then I think I might have had trouble with it that way. I took one capsule a day 3-5 days a week. In other words, I didn't take it every day and when I did take it, I took only one capsule. I tell you this for a couple reasons, one of which is NOT to tell you how much to take. I tell you what I took only for an example and to show first, that an herb can still help you whether you take it every single day or not. And secondly, that an herb can sometimes help you at a low dose where at a higher dose it will cause you trouble.

Cautions: Avoid Cat's Claw if pregnant.

Catnip (the herb)

What does it do? Used in Europe for centuries, catnip tea has been used for many ailments including colic in babies, as a sedative, for pain, and for insomnia. Catnip is an anti-spasmodic and also has mild antibiotic properties.[15] According to herbalist Michael Moore, Catnip is "An effective, if mild, antispasmodic for cramps of smooth muscle tubes, such as the intestinal tract, uterus, and the lower urinary tract."[16] Catnip has a calming effect on stomach cramps, spasms and gas. It is also considered to be a great tonic to balance the body. It is helpful in eliminating toxins from the body, as well as acting as a carminative to support digestion, relieve upset stomach, and control the symptoms of diarrhea.[17]

Why is it good for IC patients? Catnip, as long as your bladder can tolerate it, is excellent for bladder cramping and spasms. It is also excellent for the intestinal cramping of IBS. It is very good to drink around the menstrual cycle for cramps and/or any time of the month to help relax. It's also good to drink about an hour before bed to help you sleep. Catnip helps to calm nerves and makes you feel relaxed. You might also find it helpful if you're trying to quit smoking to help keep you calm or for anytime you feel stressed out.

How to use it? I used catnip in tea form, though I rarely ended up making it alone. I used to use it in combination with marshmallow root and comfrey leaf for my bladder. I also combined it with marshmallow root and raspberry leaf around my menstrual cycle to help with cramps. It also works great for relief of IBS cramping of the intestines.

Contains: Catnip is high in potassium, manganese, vitamin A and vitamin C. It is rich in iron and selenium and contains moderate amounts of magnesium and phosphorus. Catnip also contains small amounts of calcium, sodium and silicon, and some B complex vitamins.[18]

Cautions: I couldn't find any cautions for catnip.

Mullein (the herb or capsules)

What does it do? Mullein is an excellent expectorant to clear mucous from the lungs. It has been used for coughs, bronchitis, asthma, and any type of lung congestion. It is also a demulcent and an anti-inflammatory. It also has vulnerary action, meaning that it helps heal wounds or inflammation. It soothes inflammation of the throat and digestive system. Mullein helps cleanse the lymph glands and is used specifically in cases of mumps, earaches, and glandular swellings.[19] Any type of lung congestion, from bronchitis and pneumonia to a simple cold or smoker's cough, mullein is an extremely helpful in breaking up the congestion and helping to dispel it from the lungs.

Why is it good for IC patients? Mullein is great for swollen lymph glands and sinus congestion, both of which are fairly common among IC patients. Due to its mucilage and demulcent quality, it is a good soothing herb for IC patients. It soothes and strengthens mucous membranes. Mullein also helps to calm nerves and therefore helps relieve pain.[20] The potassium and B complex vitamins are also helpful to an IC patient who is much more likely to be able to tolerate this herb than taking supplements. According to herbalist Michael Moore, Mullein is "an effective tonic and strengthener of the urethra and the base of the bladder, useful in urethral swelling and congestion with incontinence."[21]

How to use it? I used mullein in a tea. I happened to buy the capsules initially, so I used to use the capsules to make a tea. This is one way to make tea from capsules. In a small fine strainer, I used to place a capsule and then put the strainer at the top of a cup of hot water with the capsule hanging out in the water. As it dissolves, the mullein is released into the water. Another way to make tea from capsules is to simply open the capsule and dump the contents into the hot water and stir. (I didn't want as much of the leftover herb in the water, so I used a strainer.) I used to add mullein to my marshmallow root tea. It can also be added to other herbs in this section, such as raspberry leaf, catnip, and comfrey leaf, or you can drink it plain.

Contains: Mullein is rich in iron. It is also high in calcium, magnesium, manganese and sulphur. It contains moderate amounts of vitamin A, C, D, and B complex. And also contains moderate amounts of potassium, sodium, and silicon, along with small amounts of phosphorus, selenium, and zinc.[22]

Cautions: I couldn't find any cautions about Mullein.

Echinacea/goldenseal (concentrated liquid with non-alcohol base)
What does it do? Echinacea and Goldenseal, though they are two separate herbs and can be taken separately, are often combined. Both of these herbs are antibiotics and both also boost the immune system. Echinacea/goldenseal has antiviral, anti-inflammatory, antifungal, and antibacterial properties. It is also used as a tonic for the lymphatic system, cleansing and reducing swollen glands. Echinacea/goldenseal also cleans the blood and clears congestion from the stomach.[23] However, it is most often used as an antibiotic.

Why is it good for IC patients? Personally, I don't recommend taking Echinacea/goldenseal in capsules. It can be much too strong of a dose for an IC patient when taken in capsules. It can also be harder on the stomach for some people that way. But, in small doses, Echinacea/goldenseal fights all kinds of infections, bacterial, fungal, and viral. It is also great for boosting the immune system so that the body can fight the infection on it's own. It is considered an excellent natural broad spectrum antibiotic by most herbologists.

How to use it? Echinacea/goldenseal is not something I would recommend taking everyday. I think it would be too hard on the digestive system, the bladder, and the rest of the body, for an IC patient. But for short-term use, I think it's a great option rather than taking synthetic antibiotics. It's a lot easier on the body than synthetic antibiotics and it boosts the immune system rather than taxing it further. Like all antibiotics (synthetic or natural), Echinacea/goldenseal should be taken for 7-10 days. And then "they" say you should take 7-10 days off. If you take it long term, some say that it will lose its effectiveness. Be careful not to take too much. A smaller dose will still work. 3-5 drops under the tongue followed by a glass of water is the way I used to take it. If you are a larger person and/or can tolerate more drops, then you could probably take 7-10 drops. (Again, I am not an herbologist, I am just offering these as examples.) I used Echinacea/goldenseal liquid whenever I was fighting an infection, whether it was the flu or a bladder infection. It's great because it works for viruses as well as bacterial infections and it boosts the immune system at the same time. I still would recommend taking acidophilus along with it though because it is, after all, an antibiotic. I also found it extremely helpful with allergic reactions. When my throat was closing up from an allergic reaction, I would put a few drops under my tongue and follow with water and within a minute, my throat would open back up.

Contains: Echinacea is high in iron, selenium, zinc, manganese, and silicon. It contains moderate amounts of magnesium, potassium, niacin, vitamin C, and E, and some B-complex vitamins. It also contains small amounts of calcium, phosphorus, sodium, and vitamin A. Goldenseal is high in iron, manganese and silicon. It contains moderate amounts of magnesium, selenium, zinc, vitamin C and some B-complex vitamins, along with small amounts of calcium, phosphorus, potassium, and vitamin A.[24]

Cautions: Avoid Goldenseal if pregnant.

Licorice Root (the herb)
What does it do? The demulcent property of licorice root eases sore throats, helps heal gastric and duodenal ulcers, and soothes mucous membranes of the urinary, respiratory and intestinal passages.[25] Licorice root not only soothes, but also provides nutritional support for the lining of the stomach and intestines. It also helps detoxify the liver

and promotes healthy liver function. Studies show that licorice root promotes the production of interferon, aids adrenal gland function, decreases muscle spasms, and increases the fluidity of mucus from lungs.[26] Because this herb nourishes the adrenal glands, it facilitates a normal inflammatory response. "Licorice root is as effective as hydrocortisone, without the side effects."[27] By nourishing the adrenal glands, licorice root helps reduce the effects of stress. It also helps rebalance the hormones.

Why is it good for IC patients? Licorice root is helpful to IC patients in several ways. The fact that it nourishes the adrenal glands and that it's helpful as an anti-inflammatory are two of the best. The mucilage quality of licorice root is also soothing to the bladder. An IC patient might also find licorice root helpful to soothe and nutritionally support the tissues of their stomach and intestines. Licorice root is considered to be a mild laxative so it can help with constipation. However, anything that cleanses the liver, IC patients would be wise to be careful with because we are so toxic and licorice root does help detoxify the liver. You don't want to de-tox your liver too fast. It will make you really sick if your body is not ready for it. In time, cleansing the liver is a great thing, but initially it will probably be too strong for your body to handle.

How to use it? I used to make it into a weak tea (so it wasn't too strong on my liver) and then I would just take a few sips. I didn't use licorice root as much as I used some of these other herbs. Though some people will probably like the taste, I really wasn't crazy about it.

Contains: Licorice Root is rich in magnesium and sodium, with high amounts of iron, potassium and silicon. It contains moderate amounts of calcium, manganese, vitamin C, niacin and B-complex vitamins. It also contains small amounts of vitamin E, B2, Pantothenic acid, biotin, and zinc, along with trace amounts of selenium, vitamin A, and Lecithin.[28]

Cautions: Avoid if you have high blood pressure, heart disease, if you're pregnant or if you have diabetes.

Chamomile (the herb)

What does it do? Chamomile helps settle the stomach, ease digestion, and gets rid of excess gas. It soothes nerves and helps with anxiety and insomnia. Chamomile "...contains tryptophan, which works like a sedative in the body to induce natural sleep."[29] It also has antispasmodic and anti-inflammatory properties. Chamomile is said to help joint inflammation and sore muscles. Added to the bath it can be very relaxing.

Why is it good for IC patients? Chamomile tea is a great source of easily absorbable calcium for IC patients. Due to its high concentration of calcium, chamomile tea is very good for soothing nerves, insomnia, cramps, and spasms. It can also be helpful to IC patients in calming the gastric system. Because it's soothing to the stomach, aids digestion, and helps with gas pains, many IC patients will probably find this herb helpful. It is also a gentle laxative.

How to use it? Chamomile is helpful in a tea to calm the stomach or nerves. It is also helpful in the bath to help with painful joints and muscles or simply to help relax.

Contains: Chamomile is high in calcium and magnesium. It contains moderate amounts of potassium, phosphorus, and manganese, along with small amounts of vitamin A, C, E, and F, iron, some B-complex, selenium, silicon, Pantothenic acid, and zinc.[30]

Cautions: I couldn't find any cautions about chamomile.

Peppermint (the herb)

What does it do? Peppermint is cleansing to the body and in this way is also a stimulant. It helps settle the stomach and get rid of excess gas. According to herbalist Louise Tenney, peppermint is not only soothing to the stomach, but also to all mucous membranes.[31]

Why is it good for IC patients? A couple of sips of peppermint tea can help get rid of excess gas and the pressure it causes. This can be very beneficial to IC patients who are bloated and feel a lot of pressure to begin with. If you can tolerate peppermint in any form (even the smell of it) it says a lot to me because it is a stimulant. In other words, it's a good sign. If you are super toxic, you will probably not like peppermint. And though it is a stimulant, it is also said to be soothing and relaxing. It can also help with bowel spasms.[32] Personally, I found it the most helpful to drink only a few sips of the tea for getting rid of excess gas and pressure.

How to use it? I would use peppermint in tea form. I'm not even sure if it's available in capsules. If you can tolerate peppermint, it can be calming to IBS symptoms and soothing to the nerves. You can combine it with chamomile if you want and sip on the tea.

Contains: Peppermint is rich in vitamin A and B complex. It is high in calcium, magnesium, phosphorus, sodium, and iron. It also contains moderate amounts of selenium and manganese, along with small amounts of vitamin C, silicon, and zinc.[33]

Cautions: Avoid if you have acid reflux or liver disease. Also avoid if you have gallbladder inflammation or gallbladder problems of any kind.

Sage (the herb)
What does it do? Sage is a purifier. It dissolves toxins from the body and is often used in herbal combinations that treat parasites and worms for example. Sage is good for the intestines, sinuses, bladder and mucus membranes. Sage is also good for nerves. Cooled sage tea makes a great gargle for sore throats and inflamed gums.[34]

Why is it good for IC patients? Many IC patients have sore throats, inflamed gums, and mouth sores and might find cooled sage tea useful as a mouthwash. Because sage is a purifier, it is great to add to healing baths.

How to use it? You can use sage in a tea, as a mouth rinse, or in the bath.

Contains: Sage is high in calcium, potassium, B1, and zinc. It contains moderate amounts of magnesium, sodium iron, vitamin A, niacin, B2 and B-complex vitamins. Sage also has small amounts of phosphorus, manganese, silicon, sulphur, silicon, sodium and vitamin C, along with trace amounts of selenium.[35]

Cautions: Avoid if pregnant.

The following are herbs that I haven't tried myself, but either would have looked into trying if I were still sick or maybe why I would be careful of them.

Alfalfa Leaf (the herb)
What does it do? Alfalfa is packed full of vitamins, minerals and chlorophyll. It is often used to purify blood, to prevent colds and allergies and to help alleviate arthritis type conditions. It contains enzymes that help in the digestion and assimilation of food. Alfalfa is also helpful to the bladder and prostate. "Alfalfa is often used to treat water retention, infection, urinary and bowel problems, muscle spasms, cramps, and digestive problems."[36]

Is it good for IC patients? I have never used alfalfa leaf tea myself, but it is something I might have tried. If your bladder can tolerate it, I think it would be a good option as a gentle cleanser of poisons and toxins from the body. Another advantage for IC patients is that Alfalfa also neutralizes the acidity of the body.[37] Made into a tea it can be alkalizing to the urine and is considered a mild and safe anti-inflammatory.[38] It's full of vitamins and minerals that are easily assimilated (versus taking the vitamins and minerals in capsule form) and this is another advantage for IC patients. Its high vitamin A content is very helpful in healing mucous membranes. I think it's an especially good option in the rebuilding stages once your bladder is mostly healed.

Contains: Alfalfa is rich in chlorophyll, protein, vitamin A, E, D, and B6. It is also rich in calcium and trace minerals. Alfalfa contains high amounts of phosphorus, iron, potassium, chlorine, sodium, silicon, magnesium, B1, B2, and B12. It has 8 of the essential amino acids.[39]

Ginger

What does it do? It alkalizes the system and is a stimulant to the digestive system. It is also a kidney stimulant that increases kidney filtration, thus helping in the removal of toxic waste from the body. Ginger stimulates circulation and sweating. It's often used as a carrier in herbal combinations because it helps move other herbs through the blood, increasing their effectiveness and absorption rate.[40]

Is it good for IC patients? I believe ginger is probably too strong for many IC patients to take internally. Because it is a stimulant and is generally not recommended for people who have ulcers, inflammation, bleeding or high fever, I don't think ginger is an ideal herb for many. However, if you can handle ginger, not only is it a good sign (to me anyway), it is also very good *for* you. It will help to cleanse and alkalize your system. I think ginger is great for external use in the bath for the joint/muscle pain that often accompanies IC.

Contains: Ginger is high in potassium, manganese and silicon. It has moderate amounts of vitamins A, C, and B complex, magnesium, and phosphorus. It also contains small amounts of sodium, iron, and zinc.[41]

Garlic

What does it do? Garlic is another natural antibiotic/anti-fungal. It kills bacteria, viruses, parasites, worms and candida. Garlic is a blood cleanser, an immune system booster, and is cleansing and stimulating to the lymphatic system. Garlic also stimulates digestion.[42] "European studies show garlic helps eliminate lead and other toxic heavy metals from the body."[43]

Is it good for IC patients? Garlic can be fairly strong and some IC patients won't be able to tolerate it. Actually, I think it's a real good sign if you can tolerate garlic. It's a great natural cleanser, antibiotic, and yeast fighter if your bladder can handle it. It's also great for clearing sinus congestion.

Contains: Garlic contains high amounts of phosphorus, potassium, sulphur, and zinc. It has moderate amounts of selenium, Vitamin A and vitamin C, along with small amounts of calcium, magnesium, sodium, iron, manganese, and some B complex vitamins.[44]

Cornsilk

What does it do? The silky tassel inside the cornhusk, referred to as corn silk, is often used as a diuretic. It's very popular in Chinese herbology and can be found in many over the counter products in Europe and the United States. Cornsilk is considered mild and non-toxic. Most herbologists agree that cornsilk is helpful in reducing pain and inflammation.

Is it good for IC patients? Personally, I would choose marshmallow root over cornsilk because cornsilk has much stronger diuretic properties. However, if marshmallow root is something you are allergic to, I think this would be a good option to try. If you are allergic to corn, I would not recommend using cornsilk.

Contains: Cornsilk contains high amounts of iron, silicon, and vitamin K. It has moderate amounts of magnesium, phosphorus, potassium, and zinc. Cornsilk also contains small amounts of calcium, selenium, manganese, niacin, and B1, along with trace amounts of sodium, vitamin A, C, and B2.[45]

Dandelion

What does it do? A blood purifier and liver cleanser, Dandelion is considered a nutritive herb that is soothing to the digestive tract and absorbs toxins.[46] It also stimulates the liver and kidneys and encourages elimination of toxins. Dandelion is said to help balance the intestinal flora and is mildly laxative as well.[47]

Is it good for IC patients? Dandelion is a fairly strong cleansing herb that I believe many IC patients will not be able to handle. In my opinion, you would have to be in the much later stages of healing your IC and have a lower level of toxicity in your body to be able to handle the liver cleansing that dandelion causes. It is also said to cleanse the kidneys, gallbladder, bladder, spleen, stomach, and pancreas, all of which, in my opinion, make it too strong for many IC patients. It is also one of the stronger herbal diuretics, though at least it is full of potassium. Where most diuretics drain the body of potassium, dandelion is actually a good source of potassium. If you can handle dandelion, it would probably be very beneficial as a cleanser, but I wouldn't recommend trying it unless you have mild IC or until you are at the later stages in healing.

Contains: Dandelion is rich in calcium, potassium and sodium. It's high in vitamin A, C, E, and iron. It contains moderate amounts of phosphorus, manganese, iron, selenium, and silicon, along with some B complex.[48]

Slippery Elm

What does it do? Slippery Elm is a demulcent and in this way is similar to marshmallow root, comfrey leaf and mullein. It's mucilage helps to heal and soothe inflamed and irritated mucous membranes. It is also said to help neutralize stomach acidity. Slippery Elm is equal to oatmeal in its vitamin and mineral content and can be used as food as well as medicine. Early settlers and Native Americans used to eat the gruel (nice appetizing word...gruel) made from slippery elm bark when food supplies were short because the herb has high nutritive value.[49]

Is it good for IC patients? I never tried slippery elm for my IC, but this is an herb that I would have probably tried had I not had such good success with marshmallow root. Slippery elm is said to be soothing to the mucous membranes of the stomach, bowel, and urinary tract. While the B complex vitamins in slippery elm would be beneficial to an IC patient, it is also what makes it less likely to be well tolerated.

Contains: Slippery Elm is high in protein and B complex vitamins. It contains moderate amounts of vitamin A and selenium, as well as small amounts of vitamin E and magnesium. Slippery Elm also has trace amounts of iron, phosphorus, potassium, silicon, sodium, and zinc.[50]

Oatstraw
What does it do? Calming for nerves, oatstraw also relaxes aches and pains, relieves body tension, and it provides nutrition for weak nerves. Oatstraw helps the immune system and is good for digestion. It is used to treat ulcers and dyspepsia and is said to give the body a feeling of "well being". Oatstraw also helps to loosen mucous from the lungs and expel it similar to mullein. It is also "beneficial for ovarian and uterine disorders."[51]

Is it good for IC patients? If nothing else is working, it can be a good relaxor, but it may also increase your awareness of your symptoms by causing some extra bloating for some people. It is good for the digestive system, like a fiber, but grainier and heavier than something like wheatgrass juice. I heard from an IC patient in Canada who swears by oatstraw tea and I promised her I would include it in my book in case it might help someone else.

Contains: Oatstraw is rich in calcium and magnesium and high in silicon and phosphorus. It contains moderate amounts of vitamin A, B1, B2, and E, sodium, iron, and selenium, along with small amounts of potassium, manganese and zinc.[52]

The following is a list of herbs that personally, I would avoid if you have IC. These are herbs that are often recommended for the urinary tract. When I talk about an herb being too strong for an IC bladder it's usually because they are either astringent or antiseptic, and/or are considered a "tonic" to tone and/or cleanse the urinary tract or bladder. It is my opinion that these herbs are generally too strong for someone with IC. However, if you are at a later stage in healing your bladder or have a milder case of IC, you may be able to tolerate some of these herbs I'm not sure. We're all different, as you know. But if you have IC like I had IC or even if you have a moderate case, I would definitely avoid the following herbs (or at the very least use extreme caution in trying).

Uva ursi –antiseptic and anti-microbial considered fairly strong
   Note: Uva ursi is sometimes called Bearberry
Juniper berries – antiseptic and diuretic
Cleavers – a mild astringent and diuretic
Buchu – a diuretic and antiseptic
Horsetail – a fairly strong astringent and mild diuretic
Usnea Lichen – an antiseptic
Goldenrod – an astringent and diuretic
Watermelon seed – a stimulant and diuretic
Couchgrass – anti-microbial, a strong diuretic
Yarrow - anti-microbial, an astringent and diuretic

Other cleansing and/or antibiotic herbs that personally, I would avoid if you have IC include the following.

Barberry (very cleansing, often used to treat cancer)
Cayenne (sometimes called capsicum) (a powerful stimulant)
Chaparral (an herbal antibiotic and strong cleanser)
Green Tea (very cleansing and contains caffeine)

I would also avoid Echinacea on a regular basis and/or Echinacea in capsule form. Echinacea/Goldenseal in capsule form can also be too strong for someone with IC.

Other herbs that are stimulants that you might also want to avoid (or at least use caution in trying), if your IC is fairly severe, are the following:
Garlic
Ginger
Peppermint
Milk thistle
Dandelion

The following herbs are demulcents that soothe and protect mucous membranes:
Marshmallow root
Aloe Vera
Mullein
Comfrey Leaf
Flaxseed
Licorice root
Oatstraw
Cornsilk

The following herbs are anti-spasmodic and help with bladder spasms:
Marshmallow root
Catnip
Raspberry leaf
Chamomile

The following herbs are alkalizing and help alkalize the body and the urine:
Marshmallow root
Comfrey leaf
Ginger
Peppermint

The following herbs are carminative and help expel gas:
Catnip
Chamomile
Parsley
Peppermint

The following herbs are anti-catarrhal and help dissolve and eliminate the formation of mucous:
Comfrey leaf
Mullein
Marshmallow root
Licorice root

The following herbs help counteract metal poisoning from mercury amalgam fillings:
Alfalfa
Catnip
Comfrey leaf
Dandelion
Echinacea
Garlic

---◆---

Other Natural Products

Essential oils can be very helpful in healing. The number one thing to know about essential oils is NOT to ingest them. They are very concentrated and highly potent. Most essential oils are not to be used undiluted directly on the skin. The only two exceptions to that rule are lavender oil and tea tree oil. They are both nonirritating and can be used full strength on the skin. You can buy essential oils at the health food store. Using natural, pure essential oils that come from plants will minimize the chance that the fragrance of the oil will be irritating to you. With IC, many of us are very sensitive to smells, especially chemical, synthetic fragrances. Breathing in the chemical, synthetic fragrances such as perfume, cologne, room deodorizers, etc. can irritate our lungs, throat, and sinuses as well as cause more symptoms in our bladders. This should not occur with natural essential oils because they are chemical free. But keep in mind that you can still be allergic to an essential oil (just like anything else). And if you're pregnant or think you might be, you might want to avoid essential oils.

Lavender oil
One of the most versatile essential oils, Lavender is one my favorites. Lavender is a very healing and relaxing scent. I used it in my healing baths because it was great for calming bladder spasms and the intestinal spasms of IBS. It's also very relaxing and smelled good. I also found it extremely helpful to put a drop or two on my finger and rub it over my pelvic area to help calm cramps, bladder spasms, and IBS spasms. Some of my IC friends like to use lavender on their pillow to help them sleep.

Tea tree oil

One of the more scientifically researched oils, tea tree oil is antibacterial, antiviral, and antifungal. It is wonderful to have around the house as a natural topical antibiotic. It is helpful to draw toxins out of the skin in a healing bath and to kill any germs that happen to be leftover in the tub after washing it. I used to add a couple drops to my healing baths. It's very strong so you don't need much. I also used it as a mouthwash (add one drop to a quart of water) when I was having a lot of problems with my teeth and gums. I know a lot of IC patients who have trouble with their teeth and gums and I think they might find tea tree oil very beneficial as a mouthwash. You can buy it in mouthwash form already, but it's a lot cheaper to make your own. Also, if you have thrush or a coated tongue (which I know many IC patients do) it can also be helpful as a mouthwash for that. Tea tree oil is also great if you happen to get cold sores. I know people who just put a dab of tea tree right on the cold sore and they say it helps it heal and dry up much faster. You can also dilute tea tree oil by wetting a q-tip and then dabbing the top of the tea tree bottle to get a small amount on the q-tip. Just gently rub the q-tip with the diluted tea tree oil on it around the inside rim of your ear. (You don't want to stick it into your ear.) This will help pull infection, wax, and/or water out of your ear.

Eucalyptus oil

Eucalyptus oil is a strong anti-microbial oil often used as an inhalant to clear the sinuses, but can also be used in the bath. I used it for both. When I used eucalyptus in the bath, I didn't have to use the tea tree oil because the eucalyptus is also antibacterial/antiviral. Eucalyptus is also good for aching joints. But for the most part, I used to open up my little jar of oil and try to inhale to clear my sinuses because I couldn't tolerate taking an antihistamine with my IC. Caution: Avoid eucalyptus oil if you have high blood pressure or epilepsy.

Rose oil

Rose oil is very soothing for nerves and aromatherapy-wise works as an anti-depressant. Rose oil is said to help calm anger. It is also useful in helping to promote sleep. You can use rose oil in a healing bath as a relaxing and calming scent. Other relaxing scents, besides Lavender of course, include frankincense, sandalwood, clary sage, and chamomile.

Peppermint oil – Peppermint oil is a stimulant. One of its more popular uses is for headaches. It can help relieve headaches if you rub a tiny dab on both of your temples. It's very strong so you don't need much at all. In fact, it might irritate sensitive skin and should be avoided if you're pregnant. Personally, I would not recommend peppermint oil in the bath for IC patients, especially those with Vulvodynia. But it is soothing and healing to the sinuses if you inhale the scent of the oil.

In general, when searching for an essential oil to use in your healing baths, it's good to use the scent that you are drawn to; the one you like the most. The five I listed are just the ones that I happened to use. But maybe you like chamomile or sandalwood or something. Go with the ones you feel most drawn to. At the same time, there are certain essential oils that I would avoid if you have IC. The following essential oils are mucous membrane irritants so you wouldn't want to use them in your healing baths, especially if you have Vulvodynia with your IC.

Allspice
Bergamot
Cinnamon
Clove
Oregano
Peppermint
Savory
Spearmint
Thyme

There are all kinds of other natural products out there. I have listed several that I feel are very helpful when healing from IC and some that I feel are too strong or should be used with caution.

Acidophilus (rebuilds, soothes, gentle cleanser)

Acidophilus is the active live culture in yogurt. Otherwise known as friendly bacteria, acidophilus helps restore health to the colon. Many people think of acidophilus only in regards to yeast prevention when taking antibiotics, but acidophilus has many other benefits. Acidophilus is considered nature's antibiotic and helps keep the intestinal tract free of unwanted bacteria. It also increases the body's ability to absorb nutrients.[1] Acidophilus not only protects against bacteria and fungus, it also detoxifies toxic substances and helps to eliminate them as well. Acidophilus actually produces some of the B-complex vitamins, which IC patients are in such desperate need of. It also helps to synthesize many of the B vitamins such as biotin, folic acid, and B12.[2] Acidophilus, taken before meals, helps digestion and eliminates undigested proteins.[3] It helps a lot with IBS symptoms and stomach problems, whether it's indigestion, gas, bloating, burning, acid reflux, or whatever.

Acidophilus is something that is naturally present in the body and should not interact with any medication or other natural products taken. It's basically like eating yogurt in that regard. It's mild, non-toxic, and helps IC patients in so many ways. Unless you are allergic to it, in my opinion, acidophilus will most likely for sure provide you some relief. Acidophilus is something I would highly recommend IC patients take (if they can) even if they are not specifically fighting yeast. I'm not sure exactly how it does it, but it seems to de-acidify the system. For me, chewable acidophilus tablets often worked better than Rolaids or Tums for an "acid" stomach. (They pretty much taste like candy so they are really easy to take.) I chewed a lot of acidophilus tablets as I was healing from having my fillings replaced. A lot of the acids/poisons were dripping down into my system and the acidophilus helped me a lot with that. It soothed my stomach and supported my intestines as I was de-toxing from the mercury. I found acidophilus helpful throughout my healing actually. I used liquid refrigerated acidophilus in my nutrition drinks and also took the capsules for a while with the anti-candida program I did.

Baking Soda (soothing, alkalizing, neutralizing, can also be cleansing)

Baking soda alkalizes acidity just like salt and therefore becomes useful to IC patients in many ways. Some doctors/people recommend a teaspoon of baking soda in a glass of water to help de-acidify the urine, but personally I think that's a LOT of baking soda/water to drink. For me, a few small sips worked just fine. You might want to try a smaller amount first and it might work out for you fine too and then you won't have to drink an entire glass full. If you are deficient in potassium or have been told to watch your salt intake, you would want to avoid using baking soda this way because it can cause a sodium imbalance. Also, drinking a lot of baking soda/water at one time can "flush" you and give you diarrhea. At the same time, drinking it too often can cause constipation.

Baking soda is a good base for a healing bath and to put on like powder after a detoxifying healing bath. In both instances it helps to absorb and neutralize the acids/toxins being excreted through the skin. You can use baking soda and water as a mouth rinse to help neutralize acids in the mouth and help with burning tongue and gum inflammation. You can use baking soda to clean either instead of harsh chemicals or after using chemical cleaners to help neutralize the chemicals. If you get a skin rash or allergic reaction, you can try a little baking soda on it to help neutralize the acids/toxins coming out of your skin. This worked great for me. Even taking a baking soda bath would do the same. If you have brand new carpeting or if there are new paint fumes in your house, for example, you can set bowls of baking soda all around to help absorb and neutralize the toxins.

Aloe Vera Juice (cleansing and soothing, especially to the intestines)

Used for centuries, aloe has been shown to have strong antibacterial properties (from the carnisyn). The magnesium lactate in aloe is a chemical known to inhibit the release of histamines and the salicylates in aloe help with pain and inflammation. Aloe is helpful to the colon and is good for chemical poisoning.[4] A juice made from the gel acts as an anti-inflammatory. But be careful of intestinal cramps if you drink too much aloe vera juice. Aloe vera can contain some citric acid, so we have to watch for that also. Another thing to be careful of if you use a lot of aloe vera is that it can deplete your body of potassium.

There are different ways to take aloe. There is freeze dried aloe, aloe vera juice, and IC Aloe. Though somewhat expensive compared to aloe at the health food store (I believe it's about $100 for a one month supply), several IC patients I know have done well with the IC Aloe. It is especially formulated for IC patients because they removed the citric acid and the ingredient that can cause intestinal upset. If you are interested in learning more about IC Aloe, you can call 1-877-345-5788 or check out the website at www.icaloe.com. If shopping for aloe vera juice, look for the "IASC certified" seal. IASC stands for the International Aloe Science Council and the seal certifies that the aloe is taken from aloe vera gel and not aloe latex.

MSM (soothing, rebuilder, gentle cleanser)

MSM (methyl sulfonyl methane) is a non-metallic element found in every cell of every plant and every animal. Not to be confused with sulfa drugs, MSM is an organic sulfur. It's a component of all living cells; a mineral that the body needs for healthy flexible cells. MSM is taken orally in capsule or powder form to help lots of different things. It helps with pain and inflammation and is good for helping damaged cartilage in the joint, ligaments, and tendons. It is also great for skin, hair, and nails. It's supposed to help with allergies by helping the body to flush out toxins and foreign substances more easily. MSM is said to coat mucousal surfaces and occupies the binding sites that could otherwise be used by challenging food allergens. It is also good for constipation. These are all reasons why MSM might benefit an IC patient. MSM is non-toxic and should be taken with Vitamin C. Since many IC patients cannot tolerate taking vitamin C supplements, Ester C or buffered C will work fine. From what I've learned, taking MSM without taking any vitamin C will greatly decrease its effectiveness.

Bovine Colostrum (gentle cleanser, boosts immune system, natural antibiotic/antifungal/antiviral)

Colostrum is an ingredient in mother's milk. Both humans and cows produce Colostrum. The Colostrum I'm referring to is taken from cows' milk immediately after the birth of a calf. It is a natural food product full of immunoglobulins that boost the immune system and kill bacteria, fungus, and viruses. Nature provides this wonderful immune system builder to help babies (and baby calves of course) to survive and grow healthy and strong. Colostrum, for those IC patients who aren't allergic to it (obviously) is an excellent natural antibiotic that doesn't kill off friendly bacteria. Unlike Echinacea/Goldenseal, for example, or synthetic antibiotics, Colostrum can be taken for longer than 7-10 days. So for those who are fighting infection and yeast on a continual basis, Colostrum might be a good choice of something to try. It's a gentle cleanser to the body that works against fungus, viruses, and parasites, all of which, in my opinion, might be involved in a person's IC. As it is gently cleansing the body of toxins/bacteria/fungus, etc., it's also providing support for the immune system and helping the body to heal. I found Colostrum extremely helpful in cleansing my body of mercury once I had my fillings replaced. I only took one a day for a while and then worked my way up to one in the morning and one in the afternoon. I could actually smell the metal coming out in the urine when I took it. I drank a lot of water each time I took a Colostrum capsule because I knew it was cleansing me and I wanted to dilute the urine as much as possible to support my bladder.

Colloidal silver (natural antibiotic/antifungal/antiviral, cleanser)

Another natural antibiotic that also kills fungus and viruses is colloidal silver. Colloidal silver is a fairly controversial natural product, which is why in *To Wake In Tears* I mentioned that I would probably recommend other things over colloidal silver. However, because I get this question a lot, I do want to make it clear that I had no problems whatsoever with colloidal silver. In fact, it worked great for me as part of an anti-candida program that I used. At the same time, I didn't buy my colloidal silver from the health food store. (I got mine from the Candida Wellness Center.) There are many brands of colloidal silver on the market and some are not as good as others (like with anything else). The ones available at the health food store typically have a smaller number of ppm's (parts per million) of silver and are often not as effective. I had read the good and bad about colloidal silver before using it, which I would recommend doing for any natural or synthetic product you are thinking of trying. And then, as I always say, do what you're most comfortable with.

Olive Leaf Extract (natural antibiotic/antifungal/antiviral, cleanser)

Olive leaf extract is known to help circulation, but more recently it is becoming popular as an effective natural antibiotic/antifungal that doesn't kill good bacteria. "Calcium enolate, the leaf's most active ingredient, is an extraordinarily effective killer of viruses and bacteria. It also keeps latent viruses from emerging."[5] Olive leaf is non-toxic, but it does cause cleansing, especially if you have yeast. So it would be wise to go slow with it to make sure you are in control of your yeast die-off symptoms and don't overdo it.

Oil of Oregano (natural anti/biotic/antifungal)

Also gaining popularity as an antibiotic/antifungal, Oil of Oregano is supposed to be an excellent yeast fighter. A few sniffs of oil of oregano is said to clear a sinus infection.[6]

Flax seed oil (soother, rebuilder)

Great for the intestines and soothing to all mucous membranes, flax seed oil is a great soother. It's soothing and non-irritating to an IC bladder and is great for IBS and/or if you're cleansing the colon. It is also a great source of omega-3 fatty acids, which are generally lacking in a person with inflammatory conditions, as well as those with immune system weakness.[7] Omega-3 fatty acids are said to be helpful in the treatment of allergies, immune deficiencies, nerve problems, and arthritis. The essential fatty acids in flaxseed oil have skin healing properties and can help in the treatment of eczema, psoriasis, or rosacea. Other sources of omega-3 fatty acids include fish and fish oils, canola oil, chia seeds, and soybean oil.[8] Like Glucosamine sulfate, Flax seed oil or fish oils are often used to replace non-steroidal anti-inflammatory medications. Both are helpful in the treatment of osteo and rheumatoid arthritis and I believe they also would be helpful to those with fibromyalgia symptoms. Essential fatty acids are needed to produce adrenal hormones, as well as to synthesize Pantothenic acid in the intestines.[9] Flax seed oil is great for constipation and soothes inflammation of the intestines and is therefore helpful to those with IBS symptoms. It is also used to treat cramps and endometriosis. For best absorption, flax seed oil is supposed to be taken with food. You can mix it into cottage cheese or yogurt or use it instead of olive oil on salads. I used to dribble it over brown rice or steamed vegetables. You can use it wherever you would use butter, but don't cook with it because it depletes it's nutritive value.

Glucosamine Sulfate (rebuilds and soothe joints)

Glucosamine sulfate is a fairly expensive supplement sold at most every health food store. Often combined with Chondroitin Sulfate, it has been used for years in Europe as a treatment for arthritis. "Glucosamine works because it provides the building blocks for new cartilage, the protective joint padding that prevents bones from scraping against each other..."[10] Glucosamine sulfates are a major building block of glycosaminoglycans (GAG's), which are proteins that bind with water in the cartilage. Instead of using non-steroidal anti-inflammatory drugs that don't heal joint damage, using Glucosamine sulfate can actually help repair the damaged joints. Some people are taking it for their bladder thinking it might help repair the gag layer. I don't know about that, but I do know that it's great for joint pain. I used it bulk form (because it was cheaper) and because, at the time, I was drinking a nutrition drink that I made in the blender, so I just threw some into that. It didn't bother my bladder at all, but as usual, that doesn't mean it won't necessarily bother yours. It provided what I would call moisture or lubrication so that my joints didn't feel like they were scraping together anymore. Most IC patients I know who have taken Glucosamine sulfate feel that it helped with their joint pain/fibro symptoms (or arthritis), but didn't notice that it helped their bladder. That was also my experience.

L-Arginine – (cleanser and immune support)

L-arginine is an amino acid (a protein). I'm not sure if this should be considered an alternative or medical treatment because some doctors do prescribe it for their IC patients (although it is an over the counter dietary supplement). Those people are told to take 1500mgs a day. As with all available IC treatments, it helps some and not others. The jury is still out on this treatment in terms of the research, but I have some guesses as to why it might work for some people with IC. Though none of the IC articles and studies that I've read have discussed these benefits, I have learned from other sources that L-Arginine helps the body when stressed by increasing the activity and size of the thymus gland.[11] The thymus gland is where much of the immune function originates. Along with supporting the immune system, L-arginine also detoxifies poisonous waste from the blood. It works with the pituitary gland and assists in nitrogen elimination.[12] I believe L-Arginine might help some IC patients by helping their body to handle stress better, boost their immune system, and detoxify and cleanse their blood.

If you get cold sores or have genital herpes virus, it is not wise to take L-arginine. The herpes virus likes to feed on L-arginine and it will cause the virus to flare up. From what I've read, you should also avoid L-Arginine if you suffer from migraines, have a kidney or liver disorder, breast cancer, or Crohn's disease.

The following is a list of natural products that personally I would avoid if you have IC. This is not to say that for certain you could not tolerate these products or find them helpful. It is just my opinion from what I've experienced that they may be too strong and/or too cleansing for someone with IC.

Homeopathic remedies
Any tincture that contains alcohol
Evening primrose oil
Grape seed extract
Green tea
Detox tea
Most every herbal combination supplement made for the bladder, such as those made for "overactive bladder" or "urinary health", or those called names like "cran support" (anything with cranberry in it) or "ultimate urinary cleanse". These are all things that personally, I would avoid.

Vitamins and Minerals and IC

As I've said before, I don't believe IC patients are absorbing nutrition properly due to a toxic colon. Even if we're eating "right" and/or taking vitamin/mineral supplements, with a toxic colon, we're not going to be effectively absorbing the nutrition and therefore it's not going to be of much help. If you have IBS (even if you're constipated fairly often for whatever reason), or if you know you have a yeast problem, for example, you can be pretty sure that you're not getting the nutrition you should be getting from your food (and/or supplements). There are many of us who are on restricted diets (e.g., the IC diet, the anti-candida diet, the gluten-free diet, the low oxalate diet, and some are even on low carbohydrate diets). On top of the lack of absorption and all the diet restrictions, many IC patients experience extra bloating and pressure from eating, which often causes more bladder pain and pressure. Often we limit our food intake just to avoid the pain. I know that's what I did. Also, we are often told to avoid certain foods and vitamins because they are known to be bladder irritants for many IC patients. For these and other reasons, it's not hard to see that we could benefit from some extra nutrition. But if our bladders (and body) can't tolerate taking vitamin/mineral supplements, then what are we to do?

As important as they are to our healing, we can't just run out and take all kinds of vitamin and mineral supplements. First of all, when the body is very toxic, taking a whole bunch of supplements is NOT the answer anyway. All it will do (most likely) is make you very sick and cause your bladder to "flare". And secondly, when you have IC and your bladder is raw (or at the very least inflamed and irritated), taking certain vitamins will most likely cause pain and further irritation. As discussed earlier, IC patients usually can't tolerate B vitamins and vitamin C in particular. They both can cause burning and pain in an IC bladder. Multiple vitamins are usually out because they contain both C and B vitamins. There are other vitamins and minerals that IC patients may not be able to tolerate as well. It's not just the B's and C, although they are the most common. Potassium is a good example of a mineral that many IC patients can't tolerate in foods or supplement form and are often told to avoid.

One thing to remember is that we can actually be allergic to vitamins and/or minerals. It is one thing that they can be irritating to our bladder and it is another thing that we can also be allergic to them. Again, this is where we are all going to be a little different. Some people ask me, what vitamins/minerals are IC safe? Just like they ask, what foods are IC safe? There is no such thing as "IC safe" in my opinion with either foods or vitamins. There are some foods and vitamins (of course) that are more than likely going to be irritants for an IC bladder, but even that is not iron clad. **We are all different in what vitamins/minerals we can tolerate and we are all different in what foods we can tolerate.** Don't let anyone tell you that you can't take a certain vitamin or that you can't eat a certain food. You very well might be able to. Granted, you very well might not be able to too. Unfortunately, trial and error is the only way to truly know for sure what we can and cannot eat, what we can and cannot tolerate bladder-wise. The most important thing is to start out by avoiding the major IC no-no's when it comes to foods and drinks (e.g., citrus fruits, juice, tomatoes and acidic foods, spicy foods and sauces, vinegar, alcohol, chocolate, caffeine) and vitamins (e.g. B complex, vitamin C). And then when you do start to experiment, it's important to go very slow. Eat only a little bit of the food or take only a portion of the vitamin/mineral supplement (or a sip of a nutrition drink). Again, this is where NAET can be very helpful. Knowing whether or not you're allergic to a vitamin or mineral before you take it can be *very* helpful. And then being treated with NAET can help your body tolerate the vitamin or food a lot more. It will "re-train" your body to recognize the vitamin or food as a good thing instead of as an allergen. Determining your allergies will help a lot, but it is not the "be all, end all" either. You can be allergic to a vitamin/food and not feel it in the bladder. In others words, you can experience other symptoms as a result of the allergy, but not necessarily in the bladder. Just as you can know for sure that you're NOT allergic to a certain vitamin or food and yet still you won't be able to tolerate it in your bladder.

Let's say that you go to NAET, for example, and find out that you're allergic to vitamin C. So you get treated for vitamin C, with NAET, and now you are no longer allergic. Does this mean your bladder can tolerate you taking vitamin C supplements? No. Not necessarily. Once you get cleared of the allergy, your bladder will not automatically be able to handle the vitamin in supplement form. Your bladder has to be healed enough to be able to handle the vitamin and even though you may have been cleared of the allergy (or tested not allergic), it doesn't mean that you can right away tolerate taking the vitamin supplement. The allergy elimination will not automatically cause your bladder to heal enough to be able to handle it. It doesn't work that way. When you get treated with NAET, as you may already know, after the 24-25 hour avoidance period, you are asked to purposely expose yourself to the allergen that you were just treated for. This is how the treatment is reinforced. Many IC patients have asked me what to do in this situation. Naturally they are afraid to take the vitamin supplement. And well they should be (if you ask me). What I did was to not take the actual supplement, but to eat or drink something that had that vitamin in it. This is much easier on the bladder and the body for an IC patient. The thing is, your NAET doctor is not going to know about this and will probably be telling you to start taking vitamin C or B complex, for example, because they will see that you need it. And they will be right, because you do need it. But you're bladder may not be ready. This is again where you will need to listen to yourself and do what is right for you and your bladder. Remember, most likely your NAET doctor is not going to know much about IC, so it's your job to know about it so that you can protect yourself.

If you are like many IC patients and already know that you can't tolerate taking vitamin/mineral supplements, then you will have to go much slower in terms of getting nutrition back into your body. And even if you are going to NAET, if your bladder is not healed enough, you will still have to go very slow. But as you begin to heal your bladder by removing sources of toxins and slowly cleansing them out of your body, soothing your bladder all the while, you will be able to get yourself to the point (and NAET can/will help) where you can tolerate taking vitamins. You might not be able to take supplements, but you might be able to drink nutrition drinks that have vitamins in them or you might be able to eat better (less of a restrictive diet) and also be able to absorb nutrition from your food better as you cleanse your colon. I gradually worked my way up to being able to tolerate various nutrient-rich whole foods and nutrition drinks with vitamins/minerals, for example. At the same time, by the time I had discovered NAET, I had already done a lot to heal my bladder. This may not be the case for many of you who are learning about NAET earlier in the process.

The main thing to do is to get as much nutrition into your body as you can tolerate without overdoing it and causing yourself more bladder pain. Herb teas are an excellent source of vitamins and minerals that are easily absorbable. They will also be soothing your bladder at the same time so therefore they will be easier for you to tolerate. But herb teas, though they *will* help and are great in the beginning stages of healing as a source of nutrition, are not going to be enough to provide you with the amount of vitamins and minerals you need to heal. It might take band-aiding your bladder in some way so that you can tolerate drinking some nutrition drinks, especially if you are in a really torn down stage. Whatever you can do to help band-aid your bladder so that you can start getting more nutrition into your body is good. It might take a while before you can heal your bladder enough with marshmallow root tea and eliminate allergies with NAET, for example, to be able to tolerate getting more vitamins/minerals. It depends on where you are with your IC and what else you are doing to get to the point where your bladder can tolerate more. Even if you prefer to go the medical route in terms of using bladder instillations, medications, or whatever, I would recommend doing whatever you have to do, whatever you are most comfortable doing, to get to the point where your bladder can handle you getting some easily absorbable nutrition into your body. Also, once you cleanse your colon and rebuild it with acidophilus, you will improve your digestion and will also begin to absorb more nutrition from your food.

If you are having success with a medical or alternative approach that is allowing you to eat or drink things that you weren't able to eat or drink before, do yourself a favor and take the opportunity to try and replenish your body with much needed nutrition. This is a time that I would experiment with some nutrient-rich whole foods such as wheat grass or barley juice, bee propolis, royal jelly, chlorella, or some form of nutrition drink. You don't want to over do it, of course, and start taking handfuls of vitamin supplements or anything. But if your bladder is somewhat under control or you're experiencing a remission or even a cover-up of symptoms, it's a good time to try getting more vitamins into your body. Many IC patients will use something like Prelief to help them be able to eat pizza, for example, which is wonderful and well deserved. Don't get me wrong. But if you have an avenue for relief that enables you to tolerate more, eat your pizza and then chase it down with some wheat grass juice or something. (I'm just using wheat grass as an example because it's jammed packed full of vitamins and minerals.) Oh...and by the way, you don't have to drink a whole big glass of wheatgrass juice or anything. Start with a couple sips and maybe work your way up to a half-cup of weak juice even. The same goes with something like Royal Jelly. Just have a small taste. You don't have to eat a whole tablespoon of it. What I'm saying here is to look for ways to sneak easily absorbable nutrition into your diet whenever possible and in whatever way you, personally, can tolerate it. If you have mild IC and from my perspective are less toxic (than someone with more severe IC) then you might be able to handle taking some vitamin supplements. And I would tell you this, if you can, I would take them for sure because I strongly believe that you need the vitamins/minerals to help your body to heal itself.

Granted, we are not all going to be able to tolerate the same vitamins and minerals, but unfortunately we are being told to avoid certain ones and that others are okay. In my opinion, this is simply not true. For example, some people say that IC patients should avoid potassium because it can be a bladder irritant. But some IC patients can handle eating bananas and avocados (which contain potassium) even though it can cause others to be reeling in pain within minutes. Some people are told that it's okay for them to take B6, just not the other B vitamins. This is not good for two reasons. First of all, just because someone says something is "IC safe" does not mean that it is. We are all different. Some people will be able to tolerate other B vitamins (B12 for example) and some people won't be able to tolerate the B6 that someone is saying is "IC safe". It's not a cut and dry thing where we can just assume that we can handle B6 because someone said it was "IC safe". And secondly, B vitamins all work together. It's not good to have a big imbalance among the B vitamins. Taking a lot of one and none of the others is not recommended. They exist together in nature for a reason. They need each other and work together, which is also why they are usually found lumped together in supplements called "B Complex". Just as we shouldn't follow a predetermined diet without determining what we can personally tolerate, it is not wise to assume that if some IC patients can tolerate certain vitamins that you will necessarily be able to.

I strongly believe that avoiding B vitamins (and/or vitamin C) indefinitely because you have IC is not a good idea. It's just going to make it harder for you to heal and most likely you will develop new and different symptoms because of the vitamin deficiencies. This is why I feel it's so important that we do other things to get us to the point where we can tolerate getting some of these vitamins into our diets or in some type of supplemental form. **Ironically, the vitamins and minerals that you have trouble tolerating are the ones you most likely need the most to help you heal.**

As I mentioned earlier, I believe that the B complex vitamins are crucial to our healing and so is vitamin C. It is my opinion that our deficiencies and intolerances to these major vitamins is intimately linked to our symptoms and to our healing from these symptoms. Understanding what these vitamins do and what can result from a deficiency in them, will help explain why I think this is the case. Also, my personal experience in healing from IC has taught me that this nutritional link, this vitamin/mineral link is extremely important. I'm not sure whether the toxicity in our bodies is what turns the switch, what makes us unable to tolerate these vitamins or whether it's a deficiency in these vitamins which sparks the inability of our bodies to process toxins out more efficiently. As Charlie always says, it's probably a combination thing.

B complex vitamins
- Essential to the health of the adrenals and the entire glandular system
- Help protect the immune response and help the body when under stress
- Help protect the nerves and nerve function
- Considered natural tranquilizers or anti-stress vitamins
- Deficiency can cause anxiety and/or panic attacks
- Essential for healthy mucous membranes
- Help to eliminate bad estrogen and toxins from the liver
- Help relieve fatigue, water retention, and cramps

131

B complex vitamins (continued)
- Help with regularity, protect the intestines and improve digestion
- Work together to nourish the thyroid gland
- Vital for enzyme reactions that control circulation, energy, hormones, and overall health

Pantothenic acid (B5)
- Essential to the body during any type of stress (physical and emotional)
- Essential to the health of the adrenal glands
- Needed for proper digestion and for metabolizing fats, carbohydrates, and protein
- Needed more during times of stress, illness or exposure to toxins
- Once in the intestines, stimulates the growth of friendly flora and is helpful in fighting yeast overgrowth and accumulations of other toxic substances, such as formaldehyde
- Necessary for the production of natural cortisone
- Counteracts the side effects and toxicity of antibiotics
- Helpful in treating the herpes virus

Pyrodixine Hydrochloride (B6)
- Involved in more bodily processes than any single nutrient
- Needed for a healthy nervous system
- Essential for proper chemical balance in the blood and body
- Very important for the proper metabolism and use of protein, fats, carbohydrates, and hormones such as adrenalin and insulin
- Necessary for the production of hydrochloric acid needed for digestion
- Necessary for the proper functioning of the thyroid so it can use iodine effectively in hormone production
- Helps to regulate the sodium – potassium balance in the body
- A deficiency can cause hair loss, skin conditions, carpal tunnel syndrome, hormone imbalances, adrenal gland exhaustion, nervousness, and dizziness

Pyrodixine Hydrochloride (B6) (continued)

- A deficiency hinders the ability to metabolize estrogen, which can result in estrogen dominance (e.g., fluid retention, bloating, tender breasts, and weight gain)
- A deficiency can result in muscle and joint pain
- Acts as a diuretic by helping to reduce water retention
- The need for B6 increases if you have a candida problem because the yeast prevents B6 from being converted into its active form, pyridoxal-5-phosphate
- Women have a special need for B6 because it performs an integral role in maintaining a balance of female hormones
- More B6 is needed if you are on a high protein diet, on cortisone or estrogen supplements, on oral contraceptives, while pregnant, and in the last two weeks of your menstrual cycle

Folic Acid (B9)

- Essential for entire nervous system
- Essential for the absorption of calcium and iron
- Essential for the formation of red blood cells and the maintenance of sex organs
- Required by the cells in the digestive tract to replicate and heal
- Folic acid is an important vitamin to help heal IBS
- Beneficial for people with restless leg syndrome, arthritis, and chronic fatigue
- Requirement for folic acid increases when under stress

Thiamine (B1)

- Helps to utilize energy from carbohydrates
- Essential for the health of nervous system
- Essential for proper functioning of digestive system
- Balanced with other B complex vitamins can help the pain of fibromyalgia
- Deficiency can result in depression or addictive behavior

Riboflavin (B2)
- Helps the body to digest and assimilate fats, proteins, and carbohydrates
- Essential for proper enzyme formation
- Essential for sodium-potassium balance
- Helps maintain good vision, and healthy skin, hair and nails
- Deficiency can impair the body's absorption of iron and weaken the thyroid
- Deficiency increases the likelihood of depression
- The need for B2 increases with critical illness

Niacinamide (B3)
- Helps the body produce cortisone, insulin, and male and female sex hormones
- Aids in healthy skin, tongue and digestive system
- Eases attacks of diarrhea
- Helps regulate blood sugar levels

Cobalamin (B12)
- Necessary to metabolize fats and carbohydrates
- Required for the body to make myelin, the membrane that covers nerves, therefore a deficiency can result in numbness or burning sensation in the feet
- Deficiency signs can include confusion, memory lapses, and depression
- Deficiency results in pernicious anemia, constipation, allergies, insomnia and menstrual disturbances
- Deficiency impairs the bodies ability to ward off bacteria and viruses
- Helps clear up hives and chronic dermatitis
- Helps correct low blood pressure that can cause dizziness
- Helps overcome insomnia
- Helps the thyroid gland work properly
- Often used to treat asthma and allergies
- Folic acid works with B12 and should be taken together

Some **things that deplete B complex** vitamin resources in the body include:

Stress and negative emotions   (especially depletes B1, B6, and B9)
Sulfa drugs   (especially depletes B1, B3, B5, and B9)
Cigarette smoking   (especially depletes B1, B2, and B12)
Estrogen   (depletes all B complex vitamins)
Birth control pills   (all B complex vitamins, with a severe loss in B6)
Excessive sugar   (especially depletes B2 and B3)
Most every pharmaceutical medication (all B complex vitamins)
Laxatives   (especially depletes B12)
Antacids   (especially depletes B12)
Heavy exercise (depletes all B complex vitamins)
Alcohol (depletes all B complex vitamins)
Excessive dieting (depletes all B complex vitamins)

Some **herbs that are rich in B complex vitamins** include catnip, mullein, licorice root, parsley, and goldenseal. Celery seed and dandelion are also rich in B complex vitamins.

Vitamin C
- Needed for healthy mucous membranes
- Necessary for the production of adrenal hormone that protect the body from stress
- Helps with the formation of connective tissue
- Deactivates free radicals
- Aids the destruction of viruses and bacteria
- Protects against mercury toxicity
- Reduces the toxicity of sulfa drugs
- Destroys toxins in the colon
- Binds foreign proteins and carries them out of the body
- Important in glandular function
- Essential element of a strong immune system
- Must be obtained daily from external sources because the body cannot manufacture it

In order for us to heal our bladders and to have healthy mucous membranes, it's essential that we get enough Vitamin C. Vitamin A is also essential to strengthen and protect mucous membranes. Both vitamins are important in healing our bladders. It's interesting to note that marshmallow root contains both of these vitamins and can be made into a soothing tea for an IC bladder.

Both B vitamins and vitamin C are water-soluble. They are not stored in our body for long periods and therefore we need a supply each day from our diets.

Some **things that deplete Vitamin C** resources in the body include:
Antibiotics
Stress
Pain medications
Cigarette smoking
Diuretics
Birth control pills
Aspirin
Cortisone drugs

Some other **herbs that contain vitamin C** that IC patients might be able to tolerate drinking in a tea include comfrey leaf, catnip, parsley, raspberry, licorice root and chamomile. Aloe vera also contains citric acid or vitamin C. Echinacea and goldenseal also contain moderate amounts of vitamin C.

Vitamin A
- Important in strengthening the cell walls in mucous membranes
- Necessary for our body to heal and repair tissue
- Helps fight infection
- Protects against the development of kidney stones
- Essential during pregnancy and lactation
- Necessary for iodine to be properly absorbed

Because vitamin A is necessary for iodine to be properly absorbed, if you have hypothyroidism (many IC patients do), then you have double the reason to make sure you are getting enough Vitamin A. But you don't necessarily want to take high doses of Vitamin A, because it is possible to overdose on it. But small doses can be very helpful in healing from IC (in my opinion of course).

Some **things that deplete Vitamin A** resources in the body include:
Birth control pills
Cortisone
Prednisone
Alcohol
Estrogen
Most drugs
Coffee

Some **herbs that contain Vitamin A** include marshmallow root, comfrey leaf, catnip, parsley, slippery elm, and raspberry leaf. Alfalfa leaf, garlic, and dandelion are also rich in Vitamin A.

Just as the B complex vitamins and vitamin C are, in my opinion, very important to healing from IC, the two most significant minerals I feel are calcium and potassium. Granted we are not all going to be the same, but I think that many IC patients could benefit from, and might possibly be deficient in, these two major minerals. Actually, with potassium, I believe an imbalance can occur either way. Where some IC patients are deficient, some may have elevated levels. It is interesting to note that calcium and potassium are both needed for the proper functioning of the adrenal glands. "Studies have shown that panic attacks and calcium deficiency tend to go hand in hand."[13]

Calcium
- The most abundant mineral in the body (which tells you right there how important it is)
- Necessary for the smooth transition of nerve impulses
- Protects the nerves and prevents toxins from irritating them

Calcium (continued)
- Necessary for the smooth functioning of the heart muscles and the muscular movements of the intestines
- Protects against a toxic environment in the body
- Needs to be taken with magnesium and ideally with a small amount of zinc
- Along with magnesium helps to relax the bowels and is good for the diarrhea and intestinal cramping associated with IBS
- Along with magnesium helps relax nerves and therefore helps to eliminate pain and ease anxiety
- Along with magnesium considered a potent sleep inducer and helpful with insomnia
- Along with magnesium considered natural chelating minerals
- Along with magnesium protect against mercury poisoning as an alkaline forming mineral
- Along with magnesium is helpful for fibromyalgia symptoms of muscle and joint pain

Some **things that deplete Calcium** resources in the body include:
Stress
Chocolate
Aspirin
Lack of exercise
Lack of magnesium
Lack of hydrochloric acid
High animal protein diet
Table salt
Excessive phosphorus

Some **herbs that contain calcium** include marshmallow root, comfrey leaf, chamomile, parsley, and raspberry leaf. Alfalfa leaf and Dandelion are also rich in calcium, but are less likely to be well tolerated by many IC patients.

Potassium

- Potassium is to the soft tissues of the body as calcium is to the bones
- Our most valuable electrolyte, crucial to life and to the functioning of every cell
- Acts with sodium to maintain normal ph levels and preserve proper alkalinity of body fluids
- Acts with sodium to balance fluids and the flow of nutrients inside and outside of cells
- Stimulates the kidneys to eliminate poisonous body wastes
- Essential for the normal functioning of the adrenal glands
- Has an important role in the transmission of electrical impulses through the central nervous system and in regulating a smooth and natural heartbeat
- Protects the kidneys, reproductive organs, and the muscles
- Good for muscle and nerve impulses
- Helps prevent panic attacks
- Helps reduce cramps and water retention
- Healing to the stomach and colon
- Prevents acidity and autointoxication

Some **things that deplete Potassium** resources in the body include:
Excessive salt in the diet
Diuretics
Laxatives or bouts of diarrhea
Cortisone drugs
Alcohol
Coffee
Cooked and processed foods
Cleansing

Sodium and potassium work very closely together and it is extremely important to keep them in balance. Along with B6 and the mineral magnesium, potassium plays a critical role in the balance of water in the body. When these three nutrients are lacking, edema can result. Severe fatigue and muscle weakness can also occur if you're deficient in these three nutrients.

I know a lot of IC patients who have intense salt cravings. Some people think it might be because our bodies are so acidic that we are naturally craving salt to help de-acidify our system. Although there are other causes I'm sure, another cause of salt cravings might be a deficiency in potassium. I know that was the cause of mine.

Some **herbs rich in potassium** include catnip, comfrey leaf, parsley, mullein, marshmallow root and raspberry leaf. Garlic and chamomile also have moderate amounts of potassium. Alfalfa and dandelion are also rich in potassium, but are less likely to be well tolerated by many IC patients.

If you're concerned that you might be deficient in these or other vitamins or minerals, there are tests that you can have done to check your levels. By the way, you can also have a test done to check the functioning of your adrenal glands. There is a saliva test called Adrenal Stress Index (ASI) where they can test the rhythm and secretion activity of your adrenal glands.

Section 6

Charts and Things

Things You Don't Have To Ingest

This section is especially for those with severe IC and/or those who cannot tolerate taking much of anything orally. For those of you who are simply too toxic and too sensitive, for those of you with so many allergies that you don't want to risk take anything new at the moment, this section contains things that you can do where you don't have to ingest anything. They are things that will help you to get to the point where you will be able to tolerate more. They are things that will help cleanse your body and rebalance your body, again, without you ingesting anything. Also, these are things that are helpful to anyone with IC and can be used easily in conjunction with the herbs and other natural products discussed in this book.

Healing Baths

There are many reasons why healing baths can be helpful to IC patients. At the same time, there are definitely some IC patients that find that cannot take baths. I have heard from some people who tell me that they get a yeast infection every time they take a bath or an IC flare up or a bladder infection for example. Possible reasons for this might be because they are either allergic to chlorine (or other chemicals in tap water), whatever they are putting in their bathwater, or maybe even what they are cleaning their tub with. I'm not sure. These are just guesses obviously. The most important thing, as always, is to do what is best for you. If baths bother you or make you worse, then I

141

would recommend NOT taking baths. (Brilliant of me huh?) If you think you might be allergic to chlorine (if pools really bother you it might be something to consider), they do make a little plastic re-usable anti-chlorine ball that you can throw in the bath and it takes out all the chlorine. You can find it at www.selfcare.com for approximately forty dollars. They even have attachments to put on the showerhead.

Our skin is our largest eliminative organ. We release toxins and waste through our skin and sweat all the time. (It's interesting to note that many IC patients have skin breakouts, skin sensitivities, skin rashes, etc.) The skin not only releases toxins, it also absorbs things. For an IC patient, a healing bath can be a great way to gently detoxify the body without ingesting anything. It will support the body's natural detoxification process, which it's already undergoing anyway in an effort to cleanse and heal itself. A slow, mild detoxifying bath can also be soothing and relaxing. (We can use all the soothing and relaxing we can get to help us heal.) An IC patient can use healing baths to relax bladder spasms and/or the spasms of IBS, to ease the burning of Vulvodynia, to help pull toxins out of aching muscles and joints and to help relax in general (maybe even before bed to help you sleep).

With IC, it is my opinion that it's really important to soothe at the same time as drawing out the toxins and also to add something that will help de-acidify or neutralize the toxins as they are being released. Baking soda is wonderful for that and I used it as a "base" in all my healing baths (except the ginger baths), but you can also use sea salts if you want. They'll work just fine. But remember, bath salts are not the same as sea salts. Sea salts are all natural where bath salts often contain synthetic colors and/or fragrances. With IC, it's wise to avoid bubble bath, bath salts, and other synthetic bath products because they will have a much higher likelihood of bothering you. Epsom salts will also work if you can tolerate Epsom salts.

A healing bath can be relaxing, soothing, and/or detoxifying depending on what you put in the bath. The following is a list of ingredients for various healing baths. These are basically the ingredients that I used just to give you an idea of how to do this. As with everything in this book, it is meant to be a starting point to help you develop your own healing baths.

How to take a detoxing and soothing healing bath:
Start with a baking soda base (approximately a 1/2 cup to a cup). It doesn't have to be exact. (I never measured once.) As the water is running, add a couple drops of tea tree oil which will not only ensure that there are no germs in your bath water, but will also help to pull toxins from your skin. Then put in a couple drops of your favorite fragrant essential oil (e.g., lavender or rose). Take a tea ball and add 2-3 pinches of comfrey leaf, a pinch of sage, and pinch of parsley if bloated. The comfrey leaf is soothing. The lavender or rose oil is great for relaxing. The tea tree oil and sage are both cleansing and purifying. And again, the baking soda will be neutralizing the acids that are coming from your skin. Stay in the bath for 5-20 minutes depending on how you feel. You'll know when you're ready to get out.

If you so choose, relaxing music, your favorite healing scents, whether natural incense or even just the scent from the essential oils you already added to your bath, and some candles will add to your healing bath experience. Besides burning natural incense and candles in the bathroom, sometimes I burned sage (the same kind of sage I was putting in the bath). I would light it and place it in an ashtray or dish and let it burn while I was in the bath.

While in the bath, it's good to have a glass of water with you to sip on and also to drink when you get out of the tub. This will help flush the junk out of you. Baking soda, used like you would use talcum powder after you get out of a cleansing bath can be very helpful in helping to absorb and neutralize the toxins/poisons that are coming out of the skin. It wouldn't hurt to have a little marshmallow root tea afterward either. (Naturally this is only recommended if you can tolerate marshmallow root tea.) The point is to do something soothing that will help support your bladder as the toxins leave your body through your urine. The water will be doing that as well, diluting your urine and therefore also supporting your bladder. It also would be good to lie down or just sit comfortably and relax for a while after you get out of the tub. In other words, don't get out and then right away start doing things. Allow yourself and your body the break.

You can take one or two of these types of baths a day if you like. You don't want to take them right in a row or anything, but you can take one in the morning and one in the evening. There was definitely a time where I was taking two a day. Go at whatever pace feels right to you. You will know when you don't need them anymore.

How to take baths for relaxing spasms of the bladder or spasms of the intestines:
Again I would start with a baking soda base (or sea salt), 2-5 drops of essential oil of lavender, a couple pinches of comfrey leaf in a tea ball. Chamomile is also relaxing in the bath if you like. (If concerned about infection, add one drop of tea tree oil.) I used to rub a little lavender on my pelvic area before even getting into the tub. This will calm bladder spasms and IBS spasms or even menstrual cramps. Stay in the tub 5-20 minutes, depending on how you feel, of course. Always follow how you feel.

What to put in the bath for pulling the toxins out of the muscles and joints:
A ginger bath is great for relieving pain in the muscles and joints (e.g., fibromyalgia). Ground ginger from the grocery store works great to dissolve in the bath. Take 1-2 tablespoons of ginger (depending on the size of your bathtub and how high you fill the tub) and stir it into the tub as the water is running. When taking a ginger bath, I only used ginger, nothing else in the tub. When you first get into the tub you can feel the ginger working because the pain in your muscles and joints will increase for a minute or two, but don't worry, it passes. And then once you get out of the tub, you will feel lots better. I would rinse off once you get out of the bath, and again, you may want to use a little baking

soda as you would talcum powder and lightly coat your arms and legs. As always, make sure to sip on a big glass of water when you get out of the tub. I only stayed in a ginger bath for about 5-10 minutes.

Many have asked me if a ginger bath would bother their Vulvodynia. I'm not sure. It didn't bother mine (though I did rinse myself off right after a ginger bath), but that doesn't mean it won't bother yours. If your VV symptoms are really bad, you might not want to risk it and might want to try another method to relieve muscle and joint pain.

Some people like to use Epsom salts in their baths. If you can handle it, Epsom salts will help to draw out the toxins, but it may be a bit strong for some people. It increases circulation and it can be too much for someone really toxic. It could give you what I always referred to as "poison rushes". Also, don't use Epsom salts in your bath if you have Vulvodynia or an open cut because it will most likely burn.

If your skin is very dry (many IC patients have very dry skin) and as long as you're not allergic, you can add plain old virgin olive oil (or all natural coconut oil) to your bath. You can even use oatmeal or you can buy Aveeno. Parsley in the bath is also good for dry skin. (You can just throw some in your tea ball with whatever other herbs you are using.)

Skin Brushing
Skin cleanses have been performed for centuries to remove toxic substances from the body using herbs, saunas, and sweat lodges. When the normal organs of elimination are overtaxed and unable to process and eliminate the toxic substances, often they are deposited in the fatty tissues just below the surface of the skin. If the skin is not efficiently eliminating wastes then there will be an accumulation of toxins in the body. Cleansing the skin is said to help in cases of severe allergies and chemical sensitivities. One way to cleanse the skin is through skin brushing. Skin brushing with a natural bristle brush (that can be found at many health food stores) can help promote healing of the organs that are burdened by excess waste, such as the bladder, intestines, liver, lungs, etc. A dry brush might be too harsh for many IC

patients, especially if you have IC related edema like I had and/or very sensitive skin. But even if you can get yourself a natural loofah for in the shower or even one of those softer mesh bath sponges that they have now in all different colors, that will work just fine to help exfoliate the skin. Avoiding sensitive areas and the head, use your brush or mesh sponge to brush in little circles beginning with your feet and up your legs, your hands and up your arms, working your way toward the heart. If you decide to do dry skin brushing, its something you would probably want to do before a shower so that you can then wash off the dry, dead skin cells. Either way, dry brushing or using a loofah or mesh sponge in the shower, skin brushing is usually recommended every other day, up to twice a day (once in the morning and once in the evening). Every little bit of help you can give your body to support it in it's natural desire to cleanse itself will be beneficial to your healing. And the skin, being the largest eliminative organ of the body, is one good place to start. This is especially so for IC patients who are much too toxic to take much of anything orally, but also for any and all IC patients to help their body cleanse itself and help their bladders heal.

Rebounding and/or exercise of any kind
Our lymphatic system does not have a pump the way our circulatory system does. It needs help to flush itself and get the lymph fluids moving. Any form of low impact exercise is going to be helpful in pumping and cleansing the lymphatic system. Doing yoga or tai chi, walking, rebounding, swimming, anything that you can do to help stimulate the lymph system (without hurting your bladder) is going to be helpful in your healing. A rebounder or mini-trampoline can be very helpful in this area, especially for those with severe IC who can barely walk because they are in such bad shape. This is the situation I was in. There was no possible way I could exercise. The only exercise I got back then was walking back and forth from the bed to the bathroom and back again. If you are at this point, a rebounder can be helpful. You can actually sit on the rebounder for a minute or two and have someone else push on it a little bit and even that little bit will help your body cleanse. As you get a bit better, you can stand on the rebounder,

keeping your feet on the mat, and just bounce very lightly. This is called the "health bounce" and will help cleanse your lymph system and strengthen all of your organs. Going very slow is fine. Even just one or two minutes at a time will be helpful. Walking, especially if you can get out there in the fresh air is also wonderful to do. Tai Chi or Yoga are also excellent if you can do them. I found swimming very helpful (mostly with my fibro symptoms), but I know a lot of people are unable to handle the chlorine and chemicals in the pool. If you have a milder case of IC and are able to exercise normally (e.g., bike riding, running) then that's great. Know that you're helping yourself to heal whenever you do it.

NAET

As mentioned previously, NAET is a great option for IC patients who are having trouble ingesting much of anything and for those who are allergic/sensitive to most everything. (I know this sounds like most of us, but those who have a more mild case of IC might not have any (or many) allergies. Or at least they might not know they do.) I think NAET is great because you don't have to ingest anything, it's painless, and it's non-invasive. At the same time, it's not a total piece of cake going through the treatments. Once treated for an allergen, you must avoid it for 24-25 hours. This can be a pain in the neck, but it's not really the "hard" part. The hard part is being able to handle the detoxing that it will cause and the symptom changes that might occur along your way to healing. It's one of those things, again, where you have to hang in there as the body cleanses itself and rebalances itself. Your bladder needs to be well enough to handle the treatments. If your bladder is bleeding, I would wait on NAET treatments until you do some soothing first. Also, I do know some IC patients who are SO toxic still that NAET will not "hold" on them. Their sources of toxins remain in place and the severity of the toxicity for them, in my opinion, makes NAET difficult. So it's not only your bladder that must be ready for NAET, some people might have to do some detoxing and soothing first. But what I hear most often is that it works great and obviously that was my experience as well.

How to find an NAET doctor:
You can go to the website naet.com to find a doctor in your area that has been trained in NAET. Or you can call the Pain Clinic in California where Dr. Devi Nambudripad trains other doctors on how to do NAET. The phone number is 714-523-0800. Once you get the names and numbers of doctors near you, you might want to call them on the phone first to ask a few questions before making an appointment.

What to ask for when you look for an NAET doctor:
Personally, I would ask how long the doctor has been practicing NAET. The person may have just been trained and have very little experience. Some may have been trained and haven't been using it, but they are still listed with the Pain Clinic because they went through the program. So I would make sure that the doctor has been doing this for a while. I would also ask them how much they charge per treatment and whether they can help you get it covered by your insurance. I would also ask whether they get right to it. In other words, do they start testing and treating for your food allergies right away? There are some NAET doctors who are also into Bioset and they don't necessarily get to the food allergy treatments until later on. It is my opinion that an IC patient needs to get right to it; to be tested and treated for the major food allergens as soon as possible and also, just as important, to get tested for all the things they are taking or planning to take. A few different IC patients I know who went to someone that they thought was an NAET doctor, but who was really a Bioset doctor. They ended up going for weeks and weeks and still they weren't being tested to see if they were allergic to the herbs or medications they were taking. If the doctor you are calling happens to be into Bioset, you can ask them if they wouldn't mind testing you for what you are taking (herbs or medications) right away because maybe some will do that for you. I'm not saying there is anything wrong with Bioset (which is an offshoot of NAET). I'm sure it is a wonderful technique and very helpful. I just believe that for IC patients, it is very important to be tested and treated for the major food allergens as soon as possible and to be tested for whatever herbs and/or medications are being taken.

You don't need to find an NAET doctor who knows all about IC (not that I think that's even possible). For example, one woman called me recently and wanted to know the name of my NAET doctor. She wanted to travel here to go to my doctor because the one near her didn't know anything about IC. I told her that I was my NAET doctor's very first IC patient. It didn't matter that she didn't know about IC. It mattered only that she knew about NAET. It was MY job to know about IC. It was my job to know not to take the homeopathic remedies or the other natural products she recommended. I'm sure they would have been wonderful, had I not had IC. And I mean no offense to my NAET doctor whatsoever by saying this because I think she's great (she knows that). But from my experience, no one out there is going to understand the extreme sensitivity of an IC patient or an IC bladder. So it is OUR job to understand. It is OUR job to protect ourselves by listening to their advice and then researching further before buying or trying anything that is recommended.

Many people have asked me how long it took me to go through all the NAET treatments. For everyone it will be different. It depends on how many allergies you have. It took me approximately 8-9 months. Initially I went once a week and then as time went on and I got stronger, I was treated for more than one allergen at a time. The last few months of my treatments I did not go very often, but there were some remaining symptoms I was having and I discovered some new allergens, so I went back and got treated for those. I haven't been back since then. I was fortunate because my treatments were covered by my insurance. I know it won't be like that for everyone. I have talked to IC patients all over the country who have tried NAET this past year. The cost of treatment for most people has been between $50-$100 per treatment. The first time usually costs more with the initial consultation and testing.

Acupressure
Acupressure is based on the same principles as acupuncture, which has been in use for centuries. Both are based on the fact that we are electrical beings that have energy pathways throughout our body. They

are both about re-balancing the body and getting the chi (or energy) to flow freely so that the body can heal itself. Acupressure is very similar to acupuncture, but there are no needles (which is a major plus if you ask me). With acupressure, you can use either a little acupressure tool or you can simply use your fingers. Acupressure, sometimes referred to as Contact Healing, is a method of contacting the electrical centers in the body in order to create that smooth flow of energy. If a pressure point is sore, it indicates that energy is leaking from it's corresponding organ, area, or gland. Holding the pressure point will seal the leak. Sometimes you can actually feel a warmth in that organ, area, or gland that you're treating as the energy flows back to that area.

There are so many great things about acupressure for IC patients. Aside from the fact that it's free and easy to do, it's available to us day and night. We are able to control how long we hold each pressure point so that we don't overdo it and we can (and should) use only the amount of pressure that we can tolerate. There are so many times where we don't feel good, where we are in pain or extremely uncomfortable and acupressure offers us a way to help ourselves and find immediate relief. It's an excellent, non-invasive way to help rebalance the body and aid the body in it's own healing process. There are so many acupressure points that we might find useful. There are pressure points to clear congestion from the lungs and from the sinuses. There are pressure points that help to relieve pain in the arms or legs, points to relieve constipation and to help with nausea, dizziness, headaches, and bloating. In fact, there are several flush points on the body that will help to release excess water and flush the lymphatic system. This is a wonderful option for those with more severe IC who are still unable to exercise in any way and who might not be able to afford to buy a rebounder. If you are in this situation or even if you would like to use another method to help your lymphatic system flush, acupressure can offer you a way to flush your lymph glands without having to do much of anything. Plus, as mentioned earlier, you'll be able to control the intensity so that you can handle the flush.

For me, if I did it too long (i.e., pressed the lymph flush points), I would feel even worse and get what I always called "poison rushes". This is how you'll know if you're overdoing it. If this happens, then you just slow down, let go of the pressure point. This also applies to reflexology (foot massages) where we also have flush points. If you overdo the foot massages, you can get that same poison rush feeling. You want to go slow with both. Even though they are both excellent ways to flush the lymphatic system, if your IC is pretty severe and you're very toxic like I was, you'll probably want to go slow. This is also one reason I preferred acupressure versus acupuncture. Aside from the needles (which are really not that big a deal actually), acupuncture can be very strong for some of us with more severe IC who are more toxic. With acupressure, you have more control over the poison rush feelings. I also had trouble with acupuncture because when I tried it my frequency was still very bad. It was a pain in the neck because the doctor had to keep removing all the needles so I could take a bathroom break and then by the time he got them all back in, naturally I'd have to go again. But if you can tolerate acupuncture, I do think it's worth a try and I do remember finding it helpful. Anything to help re-balance the body is going to be helpful in my opinion.

Below are five examples of how I used acupressure when I was healing from IC. Please keep in mind that there are entire books written about acupressure and that I'm a total layman in explaining this. I'd recommend getting a good acupressure book if you want to get into doing this. I include these examples mostly to show you how helpful acupressure can be, how we can help ourselves sometimes without ingesting anything, and how simple it is to do.

To help release excess fluid:
There are several flush points on the body, one of which helped me a lot with the "pee freeze" symptom. Gently rubbing the soft spot on each temple (at the same time) will help flush the body of excess fluid. Feel for tenderness and pain and you'll know you're pressing the right point. You don't want to press hard. Be gentle, especially with these points. Contacting this acupressure point also treats the intestines and regulates abdominal fluid.

To help clear lung congestion:
If you sit and cross your arms in front of you, reaching around to press/rub underneath your shoulder where your arm meets your back, this is an acupressure point that will help clear lung congestion. As you feel around, you will feel pain as you touch the points and then you'll know that's where to press or gently rub. You can have someone else rub or hold the points for you or you can do it for yourself.

To help clear sinus congestion:
On the back of your head on either side, down near the base of your skull and behind each ear are points for the sinuses. By gently massaging this area on the back of your head, it will help clear sinus congestion and help with a sinus headache.

To help relieve nausea:
Take your index and middle finger and hold them together. Take the inside part of both fingers and on the opposite wrist start gently rubbing making small circles. Do that for a minute on one wrist and then do the same on the other wrist. This should help relieve the nausea.

To help relieve constipation:
Another acupressure point to use on the toilet! (I'm kidding. You don't have to be on the toilet to do this.) Cross your arms in front of you and then beginning up near each shoulder, walk, with your fingers along the backs of each arm down toward each elbow. Press firmly with fingertips to where you touch the bone in your upper arm. Stop at points that hurt along the way and hold them for a minute, then continue on down the arm to the elbow. Once you reach the elbow, you can do it again. Doing this several times will send energy to the intestines and help relieve constipation.

Reflexology
Reflexology is another great way to break up toxins and flush the lymphatic system. For those still unable to exercise, this can be extra helpful in that way. It's also a great way to stimulate the immune system without ingesting anything. Reflexology is an excellent tool for

us to listen to our body. You can feel the points on your own feet, determining which ones are most tender, and then checking with the charts, will be able to determine what organs correspond with those points. Also, for the most part, a foot massage also feels terrific! I say for the most part because when you're really toxic, it will probably hurt a lot to have a foot massage. When I was really sick and my IC most severe, Charlie could barely touch my feet at all to rub them. This is one point I wanted to make sure to get in here. If you are choosing to do foot massages, make sure you don't overdo it. You don't have to go nuts and rub your feet three times a day or anything. Really, you don't want to overdo anything I talk about in this book. Moderation, gentleness, slowness...these are often the keys to getting better when you have IC.

Again, there are entire books written about reflexology and I can only touch on it here. However, in one sense, with reflexology, you don't have to be some big huge expert in it either. Just having a chart and knowing some basic things, you can get started right away. Therefore, I thought it would be really helpful to include reflexology charts for the hands and feet so that you could get started without having to go out and buy another book. The things that I think are important to know ahead of time are as follows.

1) Use some type of lotion or oil (in other words, don't rub your feet without lubrication).
2) Drink plenty of water (and/or maybe even some marshmallow root tea for example) after a foot massage.
3) Do not use fingernails!
4) Use only a light touch and don't exceed ten minutes.
5) It's often recommended that when chronically ill that you only do foot massages three times a week. To be honest, I did them a little more often than that. It's important to go by how you feel and just remember not to overdo it. A foot massage can be very helpful if you're having bladder cramping with "pee freeze". It will help relax your body and help you initiate the stream.

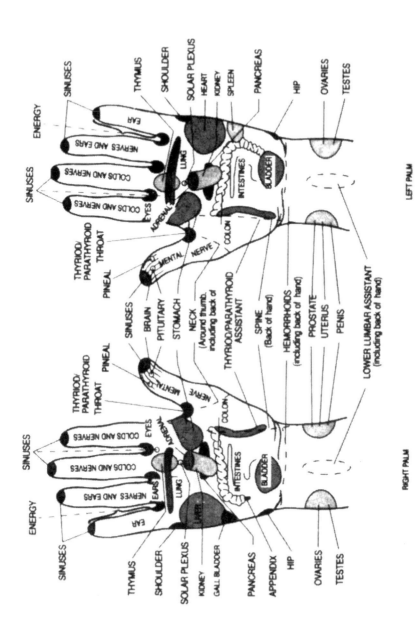

ENERGY

SINUSES

THYMUS

SHOULDER

SOLAR PLEXUS

HEART

KIDNEY

SPLEEN

PANCREAS

HIP

OVARIES

TESTES

EAR

NERVES AND EARS

COLDS AND NERVES

COLDS AND NERVES

EYES

ADRENAL

LUNG

INTESTINES

BLADDER

COLON

SINUSES

THYROID/
PARATHYROID
THROAT

PINEAL

MENTAL NERVE

SINUSES

BRAIN

PITUITARY

STOMACH

NECK
(Around thumb,
including back of
hand)

THYROID/PARATHYROID
ASSISTANT

SPINE
(Back of hand)

HEMORRHOIDS
(including back of hand)

PROSTATE

UTERUS

PENIS

LOWER LUMBAR ASSISTANT
(including back of hand)

LEFT PALM

THYROID/
PARATHYROID
THROAT

PINEAL

MENTAL
NERVE

COLON

SINUSES

COLDS AND NERVES

COLDS AND NERVES

NERVES AND EARS

EYES

ADRENAL

LUNG

LIVER

INTESTINES

BLADDER

EARS

EAR

ENERGY

SINUSES

SINUSES

THYMUS

SHOULDER

SOLAR PLEXUS

KIDNEY

GALL BLADDER

PANCREAS

APPENDIX

HIP

OVARIES

TESTES

RIGHT PALM

154

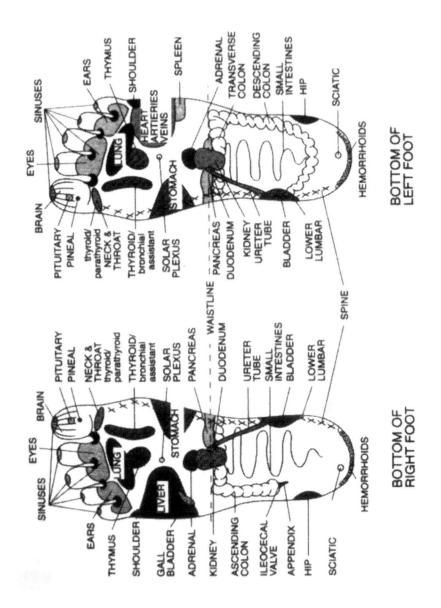

EYES
SINUSES
BRAIN
EARS
THYMUS
SHOULDER
PITUITARY
PINEAL
thyroid/
parathyroid
NECK &
THROAT
THYROID/
bronchial
assistant
SOLAR
PLEXUS
STOMACH
LUNG
HEART
ARTERIES
VEINS
SPLEEN
ADRENAL
TRANSVERSE
COLON
DESCENDING
COLON
SMALL
INTESTINES
HIP
SCIATIC
PANCREAS
DUODENUM
KIDNEY
URETER
TUBE
BLADDER
LOWER
LUMBAR
WAISTLINE
HEMORRHOIDS
SPINE

**BOTTOM OF
LEFT FOOT**

PITUITARY
PINEAL
NECK &
THROAT
thyroid/
parathyroid
THYROID/
bronchial
assistant
SOLAR
PLEXUS
PANCREAS
DUODENUM
URETER
TUBE
SMALL
INTESTINES
BLADDER
LOWER
LUMBAR
BRAIN
EYES
SINUSES
EARS
THYMUS
SHOULDER
GALL
BLADDER
ADRENAL
KIDNEY
ASCENDING
COLON
ILEOCECAL
VALVE
APPENDIX
HIP
SCIATIC
LUNG
STOMACH
LIVER
HEMORRHOIDS

**BOTTOM OF
RIGHT FOOT**

155

Meditation
Meditation is a deep form of relaxation and is very healing to the body. I believe it's an excellent thing for an IC patient to get into the habit of doing, especially because most of us are under so much stress. However, meditation, initially, will probably be difficult. I know it was for me. My frequency got in the way of being able to sit or lie down for long enough and the pain made it extremely difficult to relax or concentrate. I bought meditation tapes to help me learn to meditate. I found it much easier to listen to the voice on the tape telling me what to do, rather than just trying to meditate on my own. I think I would have just pulled all of my hair out from frustration had I tried to meditate on my own back then. Even if you find meditation difficult or you're just not into that sort of thing, any form of deep relaxation will do. Maybe you have a hobby that helps you relax. Maybe petting your dog or cat is relaxing for you. Maybe you would rather do yoga, tai chi, or some other form of martial arts. Anything that will help you relax is going to be beneficial to your healing. At worst, try to take a nap during the day to slow down your body and help it to heal. Using creative visualization and picturing yourself healthy while you're meditating or just before you go to sleep is also very helpful.

Massage and/or self-massage
Any form of massage will help to move the lymph system and break up toxins. If you are fortunate enough to have a loved one willing to give you massages or can afford to pay someone for them, they can help with fibromyalgia pain and can also help cleanse your body of toxins. Make sure to drink plenty of water after you get a massage. If you are unable to have someone else give you a massage, there is nothing wrong with self-massage. Actually, some people with fibromyalgia (or IC related edema) might find it too painful to have someone else give them a massage. That's how I was for a while. When I was all swelled up I couldn't even do self massage, let alone have someone else touching me. If you are at that point you might want to hold off on the massages (obviously). Self-massage can be good because you can go slow and not use a lot of pressure.

Breathing

I saved the most important one for last. I don't know if I can stress enough, the importance of breathing. Obviously, without breathing we can't live, so it's extremely important that way. But breathing not only sends oxygen to our cells, it is also very important for other reasons. Breathing helps pump the lymphatic system and is cleansing to the body. It helps us relax and "slow down" which is extremely important and helpful to healing. When my IC was severe, I could barely breathe. Taking deep breathes, laughing hard, coughing or sneezing, all caused a lot of pain. When I was at that point, I was breathing really shallow, short breathes or even holding my breath for long periods so as not to cause more pain. I didn't even realize it for a long time until a friend pointed it out to me. Take a moment to notice your breathing. If you're not doing much of it, think about trying to consciously change that as much as possible. Meditation or yoga will help with breathing also. One other thing I realized (actually Charlie realized it for me) is that when I got scared, upset, really stressed out or something, I would barely breathe and this would make me not feel good (or should I say, this would make me feel even worse). It is during those times, or times when the pain is really bad that we need to remember to breathe. It will help with the pain (just like in Lamaze), as it will help us relax, and send much needed oxygen into our body.

Quick Reference Chart

Things that are soothing
Marshmallow root (soothing to mucous membranes)
Mullein (soothing to mucous membranes)
Comfrey leaf (soothing to mucous membranes)
Aloe Vera (soothing to the intestines and mucous membranes)
Acidophilus (soothing to the stomach and intestines)
Flax Seed Oil (soothing to the intestines and any inflammation)
Glucosamine Sulfate (soothing to the joints)
Vitamin E (soothing to mucous membranes)
Licorice root (soothing to mucous membranes)
Slippery elm (soothing to mucous membranes)

Things that are cleansing to the body
Removing a source of toxin
Water is a very, very gentle purifier to the body
Menstrual cycle
Exercise/Rebounding
NAET
Acupuncture and acupressure
Reflexology
Massage
Certain types of herbal baths
Colostrum
Colloidal Silver
Olive leaf extract
Oil of oregano
Garlic
Ginger

Things that are antibiotic/anti-fungal/antiviral
Echinacea/Goldenseal
Colostrum
Colloidal Silver
Olive Leaf Extract
Oil of oregano
Tea Tree Oil (don't ingest – external use only)
Garlic

Things that might help bladder spasms
Marshmallow root tea
Marshmallow root tincture
Catnip tea (catnip with marshmallow root)
Raspberry leaf tea
Chamomile tea
Heating pad
Lavender oil (a little rubbed over the pelvic/bladder area)
Breathing and relaxing the body
A relaxing herbal bath with lavendar or chamomile

Things that might help when you can't sleep
Catnip tea
Chamomile tea
Sleep meditation tape
Foot massage or any type of massage
Lavender oil in the bath before bed
Lavender on your pillow
Calcium and magnesium an hour before bed
Getting some form of exercise during the day

Things that might help with IBS
Acidophilus
Calcium and magnesium
Rolaids/Tums (which are really calcium/magnesium in another form)
Flax Seed Oil
Marshmallow root in capsule form
Cat's Claw (cleansing to the colon and boosts immune system)
Lavender oil rubbed over belly to calm spasms
Wheat grass juice
Digestive enzymes
Catnip and raspberry leaf tea

Things that might help with Fibromyalgia
Glucosamine sulfate (soothing to the joints)
MSM
Exercise (swimming, yoga, walking...low impact exercise)
Ginger baths
Massage or self-massage
Reflexology
Acupressure points to relieve muscle and joint pain
Determine and eliminate allergies with NAET
Calcium and magnesium

Things that might help with Vulvodynia
Baking soda in the bath or with water on a washcloth
Low oxalate diet helps some people
Calcium Citrate (taken orally)
Aloe vera gel on the vulva area
Vitamin E oil on the vulva area
Rinsing after urinating using a small quirt bottle

Things that might help sore tongue, sore/inflamed gums, mouth sores and/or blisters
Black walnut in a non-alcohol tincture (either a glycerin tincture or black walnut oil) will help to nourish and heal sores in the mouth and throat. This herb may be helpful to IC patients who, like me, have had to deal with blisters in the mouth and throat, receding gums and/or sore, inflamed gums. I had good success using black walnut. I rubbed it on my gums, waited a minute and then rinsed it out. Be careful that it doesn't discolor your teeth though. That happened to me temporarily. Baking soda, being a natural teeth whitener fixed that problem for me. Because I was constantly rinsing my mouth with baking soda and water to help neutralize the acid/poisons back when my teeth and gums were really bad, it just naturally whitened my teeth. I think my teeth are whiter now than before I got sick!

Rinsing the mouth with baking soda and water will help neutralize the acids in the mouth and can help with burning and/or sore tongue.

Using tea tree oil toothpaste or one drop of tea tree in a quart of water as a mouthwash will fight infection and help ease the pain of sore gums.

Rinsing mouth with cooled marshmallow root tea will help soothe inflamed gums and help to heal mouth sores and blisters. Cooled sage tea is also a good mouth rinse.

From what I have learned, hydrogen peroxide can be rough on the gums if used too often. I would also recommend NOT using regular mouthwashes, which typically contain chemicals and/or alcohol.

Other things I found helpful to have around:
Heating pad(s)
Loose, comfortable clothing that doesn't press on the bladder/pelvic area
Aloe Vera toilet paper
A small squirt bottle for warm water to help initiate the urine stream
(A large squirt bottle to squirt annoying family and friends that say stupid things like "well you look okay" or "so...are you better yet?")
A tea ball for the bath and/or for making herb tea
A comfy bath pillow and cushioned bath matt
A cool washcloth for the back of the neck (well you don't have to keep it cool ALL the time)
Small icepacks (great for Vulvodynia) and large icepacks if you have swelling
Meditation tapes
Yoga or tai chi tapes
Coconut Oil (or whatever kind you prefer) for self-massage or preferably for someone else to massage you with
A gratitude journal to write in to remind us that we still have things to be grateful for even though we are suffering with IC

"You are braver than you believe, stronger than you seem, and smarter than you think."
- Christopher Robin

Section 7

Key Things to Remember

As you can see, there are no easy answers. There are no promises of a miracle cure or something that sounds "too good to be true". What I am here to tell you is that I believe the "cure" for IC is a long hard path. It is a path that has uncertainties and pain along the way, a path that may have you, at times, taking one step forward, two steps back. It's a path that will be different for everyone, one that you will have to figure out for yourself (because only you can). What my books hopefully "show" you is that it IS possible to get better, that you CAN and that you WILL find your way. If you get to the root of the problem, if you remove whatever sources of toxins might be affecting you, if you soothe, cleanse and then rebuild and rebalance your body, you CAN heal. It matters not how long you've had IC, how old you are, how damaged your bladder or how severe your IC. There truly is hope for all who read these words. This I know for sure.

Remember…just because "they" say there is no cure, it does not mean that you can't get better. It only means that "they" haven't figured it out yet. That's all it means. It does NOT mean you can't get better.

As with any chronic "incurable" disease, the word "cured" usually gets everyone up in arms. It's just one of the many reasons why, personally, I never use that word. It gets people upset and understandably so. No one can believe it when someone says they are cured of IC. Other IC patients will usually say one of two things. Either 1) the person must not have had IC to begin with, or 2) it's probably just a remission and the person just "thinks" they are cured. I know one woman who had

165

fairly severe IC and got better doing some different alternative treatments. She went to her "IC expert" doctor who she had been seeing for several years (as she was getting worse and worse) all excited to share with him how she got better and what she did, etc. He didn't want to hear a word about it. He brushed her off and as he walked away and out of the room...do you know what he said? He said, "You'll be back. You'll see. You'll be back." (By the way, this was well over 3 years ago and she is still doing wonderfully.) There are even some doctors who refuse to believe that we can get better. It is so ingrained into us that IC is "incurable".

I've also seen this happen several times over the past 6 years in our AOL IC support group. There have been IC patients who have come along and shared that they were cured of their IC by doing such and such a treatment, from taking colloidal minerals or eating cloves of garlic to being healed by a psychic healer or taking antibiotics. I remember thinking...I find it hard to believe that someone could just take one thing, like minerals for example, and get better from IC. I found it hard to believe that this person had the same IC as I had. Well the truth of the matter is that we don't all have the same IC. And where one thing might work for one person, it might not work for another. The truth is that for some people, it might only take one thing to put them back into balance. It might only take one thing to help cleanse out the bad stuff, for example, and put their body back on track. But the real question is...why are we so quick to not believe them? And why do some people find it so upsetting that other IC patients might find some hope in that person who got better? Are we afraid that others might think we aren't trying hard enough? Are we jealous that they are better and we are not? Or do we just believe that it's ALWAYS going to come back and that "remission" is the ONLY thing possible? Why are we not instead, happy to know that there are actually people out there who get better? I'm not sure what the answers are, but I do think fear has something to do with our response.

For me...I get this question all the time. People ask me all the time if I am cured because of *To Wake In Tears*. They want to know if I consider myself cured and if I am "still cured" (is the way many put it). I call what happened to me recovery. (Actually, it didn't "happen" to me, I worked my butt off to get here.) I never say that I am cured. I didn't say it in *To Wake In Tears* and I never say it in real life either. First because there wasn't just one thing that I did or one thing that I took that "cured" me from IC. "Cured" implies, to me, that some "thing" cured me. This was not the case for me. I got better gradually, treating my entire body, and over time, my entire body healed. Not just my bladder, but also my fibro, IBS symptoms, etc. Just as I got them all together, they all got better together. I didn't experience flares and remissions with my IC. I just got IC and had it. I never had that wax and wane experience that some people have. As I said, I got better gradually over time. It was not some kind of spontaneous thing nor was it one specific thing I did.

"Cured" also implies that it can never come back. I highly doubt that anyone who feels cured of IC or who feels like they recovered (like myself for example) doesn't realize that if they were to "not take care of themselves" that their IC might come back. For example, I am well aware that I need to be more conscientious in taking care of myself than I used to be before I ever got IC. I need to make sure I get the vitamins and minerals I need to STAY healthy. I need to make sure that I don't start smoking again (I can't imagine that I would) or start eating a bunch of garbage food and not taking care of myself. (Naturally I have no intention of ever having mercury put into my mouth again.) Obviously, I plan to take care of myself. And because I can eat and drink whatever I want without fear of IC symptoms, because I can have sex without pain, because I am now a healthy person with a strong immune system, I do consider myself "recovered". It would take a lot of effort on my part to get THAT full of poison and toxins again for my IC to return the way it was and I honestly don't see that happening. But naturally I must admit that there is always the chance that my IC could return in some form or another. To be honest, I try not to worry about that, knowing that I am taking good care of myself and also knowing that at least I'll know what to do if that happens.

As I've said before, none of our paths will be alike. None of our bodies will have the exact same symptoms. None of us are going to have the exact same sources of toxins to our bodies. None of us will be able to tolerate the exact same treatments or to do things in exactly the same order. This is why it is so important for us to take control of our healing, to look to our own body and our own circumstances, and to do what we feel most comfortable doing after researching as much as we can.

I'm not going to lie to you. The more toxic you are, the longer you've had IC, the longer it will take for you to get well (in my opinion of course). But you CAN get well. It IS possible. I am not an anomaly. I am not the only person with IC who has gotten better. But we are not so easy to find. I think that most people who get better go on with their lives and we simply don't hear much from them. They don't attend IC support group meetings or spend time posting to IC message boards on line. But they are out there. I know several of them. They do exist and that's the important thing to remember. I am also not an anomaly in terms of my views of IC. There are other people who recognize that IC patients have a toxic body. In fact, there are doctors out there who believe that many of these chronic illnesses are rooted in the toxic body. These are not new ideas I'm talking about here. And these are not out of control suggestions I'm making either. It's not outrageous to consider removing sources of toxins to our body. It's not "out there" to suggest that we soothe our bladders with something non-toxic and natural. It's not insane to consider boosting our immune system and getting more nutrition into our bodies. What I'm talking about here in this book is not some extreme, radical approach. Instead it is a soothing, gentle, slow, and in my opinion, safer approach than most of the medical treatments that are currently being used. In fact, going slow and being gentle with what we are taking and with our bladders (and body in general), to me, is a very important key thing to remember along your healing path.

Remember to be gentle with yourself in terms of what you are taking and what you are doing to your body. Your body is already under a lot of stress right now. That's why you have symptoms. So you will want to be gentle with yourself in terms of the things you are taking, how much of them you are taking, how many things you are taking, and what you are doing to your body. If you find an herb or natural product that helps you, for example, don't take tons of it or overdo it by taking it for months and months on end without taking a break. It's important to, at times, re-evaluate your situation and decide whether you even still need that particular herb or product anymore, for example. Just as you don't want to take multiple natural antibiotics, you also don't want to take multiple cleansers. Remember, it's not necessary to cleanse really hard or really fast. Take it easy on yourself as you go through the cleansing process and make sure to soothe all along the way. Whether it be invasive procedures, surgery, medications, or natural products or treatments that are too strong, all of these are going to put further stress on your body. Be gentle with yourself. Be gentle with your body.

Remember to be nice to yourself just in general. This is something I'm STILL working on, by the way. I know so many IC patients who aren't nice to themselves. We push ourselves and do for others and pretend we're not sick. Often we're told that the problem is just in our bladder so we don't feel we have the right to act like we're sick. Plus, many of us don't look sick so that's probably another reason. For now, accepting your limitations and **taking care of yourself first** is the smart thing to do, the healing thing to do. As you know, certain physical activities are going to make you feel worse and cause you to suffer more. My best advise, something I had to learn the hard way and did "wrong" nearly the entire time I was healing...don't do these things that are going to hurt you just to please others. Whether it's riding a long distance (or even a short one) in the car, whether it's having sex with your spouse, whether it's standing in the kitchen cooking dinner, whether it's exposing yourself to cigarette smoke, perfume, or paint fumes, whatever it is that you know is going to make you feel worse.... DON'T DO IT. I know this advice might sound stupid and pretty obvious, but I know so many of us that do all these things and more because we don't think people understand that it really HURTS, that we really ARE SICK, that we really are unable to do these things without causing ourselves to suffer even more. If they don't care enough to understand enough, then YOU will have to care enough. You will have to care enough about yourself to not cause yourself more pain and suffering than you are already experiencing right now. And if you don't care enough about yourself to do that right now...START. If you want to get better, I'd start right away.

As much as you can remember to and are able, another key thing to remember while you are getting better is to rest, to breathe, and to relax. I talked about having to feel your way through your healing and having to trust and act on the feelings you are experiencing. I meant that in many ways and this was one of them. When you are tired, you will need to rest. When you're stressed out, you will need to take time to relax and breath and meditate. Allow yourself the luxury of taking care of yourself, of putting yourself first, of making your healing a priority. Understanding the role that stress is playing in your IC is very important. Understanding that it is not your "fault", but that you are probably deficient in certain key vitamins and minerals that your body NEEDS to be able to physically handle stress. This is why it's so important to eliminate as much stress as possible while you are trying to heal. Until your body heals enough for you to be able to get these vitamins and minerals back into it, you would do best to avoid as much stress as possible, both physical and emotional.

Remember...if you get stuck, if you hit a plateau in your healing, look to your sources. Look to see what else is causing toxins in your body or what else is stressing you physically or emotionally. Look to see what vitamins and minerals you are lacking as well. All of these things will lead you to answers of what direction to go in next. Always know that you have more options.

You can do this! But it's not easy. I would never say that it's easy. In fact, it's a lot of hard work. Healing from IC is not a pleasant experience. Healing can mean that you have to make some changes in your life. Maybe you have to get away from toxic relationships in your life where you are being emotionally/verbally abused. You might have to quit smoking and change your eating habits. You may have to spend the time and the money to have NAET treatments done or to have your fillings replaced. You might have to take time out of your life right now, to rest and heal, so that in the future you can live NORMALLY again. You might have to quit working or change jobs or eliminate various stressors in your life so that you can give your body a chance to heal. None of these things are easy. And to top it all off...it's not easy physically either. You will have cleansing reactions, healing crisis, whatever you want to call them, on your way to getting better. You will have doubts and fears and you will have physical pain and discomfort. I'm not saying that you won't. I know I certainly did. And there are also times you might have a setback or at least feel like you are having one (because sometimes its hard to tell). And through all this you will need to believe that what you are doing is right; that how you are approaching your IC and your healing is for the best. That if you just hang in there and be patient, with yourself and with your body, that you will be able to bring it back into balance. You will be able to heal. It's not going to happen overnight. It took me a few years to get better, not months. But I was a severe case, so keep that in mind. Also keep in mind that I did get better and better along the way. The less severe your IC, the less toxic you are, the fewer sources of toxins you have to get rid of, and the less time you have been sick, the faster it will be for you to get better.

Get into your healing! Make lists of ideas of things to look into, do some research to make sure you're not hurting yourself, find a forum to talk to other IC patients, whether locally or on line, make a list of supplies and treat yourself to them, whether it be a comfy bath pillow for your healing baths, some herbs and essential oils, a healing meditation tape, or some books on the mind/body/spirit connection. Start believing that you can get well and get into it!

If I could go back in time (like in the Back to the Future movie) and talk to myself when I was in the midst of my horrid experience with IC, the biggest most important thing that I would want to tell myself is to try not to be so afraid; to have faith and believe that I would get well. I talked about this in *To Wake In Tears* and I feel the need to say it again because it is SO important to healing. BELIEVE YOU WILL GET WELL and you will help to create that reality.

171

Endnotes and References

Endnotes for Section 1

[1] Tenney, Louise, M.H. *The Encyclopedia of Natural Remedies.* Pleasant Grove, Utah: Woodland Publishing, Inc., 1995: 193.

[2] Ibid., p. 195.

[3] Krohn, Jacqueline, MD, Taylor, Frances A., MA, and Proseer, Jinger, LMT. *The Whole Way to Natural Detoxification: The complete guide to clearing your body of toxins.* Hartley & Marks Publishers, 1996: 141.

[4] Tenney, Louise, M.H. *The Encyclopedia of Natural Remedies.* Pleasant Grove, Utah: Woodland Publishing, Inc., 1995: 193-4.

[5] Ibid., 193.

[7] Ibid., 157.

[8] Krohn, Jacqueline, MD, Taylor, Frances A., MA, and Proseer, Jinger, LMT. *The Whole Way to Natural Detoxification: The complete guide to clearing your body of toxins.* Hartley & Marks Publishers, 1996: 134-5.

[9] Ibid., 135.

[10] Stein, PC, Torri, A, Parsons, CL.. *Elevated urinary norepinephrine in interstitial cystitis.* Urology, 1999, June: 53(6): 1140-1143. Department of Surgery, University of California San Diego Medical Center, USA.

[11] Tenney, Louise, M.H. *The Encyclopedia of Natural Remedies.* Pleasant Grove, Utah: Woodland Publishing, Inc., 1995: 157.

[12] Ibid., 186.

[13] Ibid., 186.

[14] Alagiri, M., Chottiner S., Ratner, V., Slade D., Hanno PM *Interstitial cystitis: unexplained associations with other chronic disease and pain syndromes.* Urology, 1997, May: 49 (5A Suppl):52-57 Department of Urology, Temple University School of Medicine, Philadelphia, PA.

[15] Tenney, Louise, M.H. *The Encyclopedia of Natural Remedies.* Pleasant Grove, Utah: Woodland Publishing, Inc., 1995: 258.

[16] Ibid., 258.

[17] Keay, S., Warren, J.W., et al. *Antiproliferative activity is present in bladder but not renal pelvic urine from interstitial cystitis patients.* The Journal of Urology, 1999, October, 162(4): 1487.

[18] Mulholland, S. G., Byrne, D.S., et al., *The urinary glycoprotein GP51 as a clinical marker for interstitial cystitis.* The Journal of Urology, 1999, June 161: 1786.

Endnotes for Section 4

[1] Moore, Michael *Herbs for the Urinary Tract: Herbal relief for kidney stones, bladder infections and other problems of the urinary tract.* New Canaan, Connecticut: Keats Publishing, Inc., 1998: 60.

[2] Tenney, Louise, M.H. *Health Handbook.* Pleasant Grove, Utah: Woodland Books, 1994: 190.

[3] Tierra, Lesley, L.Ac. *Herbalist The Herbs of Life: Health & Healing Using Western & Chinese Techniques.* Freedom, California: The Crossing Press, 1992: 59.

[4] Williams, Jude C., MH, ND *Nature's Gentle Cures: Safe and Effective Healing Therapies.* New York, New York: Sterling Publishing Co., Inc., 1997: 125.

[5] Tenney, Louise, M.H. *Health Handbook.* Pleasant Grove, Utah: Woodland Books, 1994: 167.

[6] Tierra, Lesley, L.Ac. *Herbalist The Herbs of Life: Health & Healing Using Western & Chinese Techniques.* Freedom, California: The Crossing Press, 1992: 59.

[7] Castleman, Michael *The Healing Herbs: The Ultimate Guide to the Curative Power of Nature's Medicines.* New York: Bantam Books, 1991: 409.

[8] Tierra, Lesley, L.Ac. *Herbalist The Herbs of Life: Health & Healing Using Western & Chinese Techniques.* Freedom, California: The Crossing Press, 1992: 74.

[9] Tenney, Louise, M.H. *Health Handbook.* Pleasant Grove, Utah: Woodland Books, 1994: 193.

[10] Tenney, Louise, M.H. *The Encyclopedia of Natural Remedies.* Pleasant Grove, Utah: Woodland Publishing, Inc., 1995: 195.

[11] Tenney, Louise, M.H. *Health Handbook.* Pleasant Grove, Utah: Woodland Books, 1994: 193.

[12] Ibid., 198-9.

[13] Williams, Jude C., MH, ND *Nature's Gentle Cures: Safe and Effective Healing Therapies*. New York, New York: Sterling Publishing Co., Inc., 1997: 23.

[14] Tenney, Louise, M.H. *Health Handbook*. Pleasant Grove, Utah: Woodland Books, 1994: 199.

[15] Ibid., 44.

[16] Moore, Michael *Herbs for the Urinary Tract: Herbal relief for kidney stones, bladder infections and other problems of the urinary tract*. New Canaan, Connecticut: Keats Publishing, Inc., 1998: 50.

[17] Castleman, Michael *The Healing Herbs: The Ultimate Guide to the Curative Power of Nature's Medicines*. New York: Bantam Books, 1991: 149.

[18] Tenney, Louise, M.H. *Health Handbook*. Pleasant Grove, Utah: Woodland Books, 1994: 163.

[19] Ibid., 191.

[20] Tenney, Louise, M.H. *The Encyclopedia of Natural Remedies*. Pleasant Grove, Utah: Woodland Publishing, Inc., 1995: 206.

[21] Moore, Michael *Herbs for the Urinary Tract: Herbal relief for kidney stones, bladder infections and other problems of the urinary tract*. New Canaan, Connecticut: Keats Publishing, Inc., 1998: 62.

[22] Tenney, Louise, M.H. *Health Handbook*. Pleasant Grove, Utah: Woodland Books, 1994: 191.

[23] Tenney, Louise, M.H. *The Encyclopedia of Natural Remedies*. Pleasant Grove, Utah: Woodland Publishing, Inc., 1995: 195.

[24] Tenney, Louise, M.H. *Health Handbook*. Pleasant Grove, Utah: Woodland Books, 1994: 171, 180.

[25] Tierra, Lesley, L.Ac. *Herbalist The Herbs of Life: Health & Healing Using Western & Chinese Techniques*. Freedom, California: The Crossing Press, 1992: 68.

[26] Williams, Jude C., MH, ND *Nature's Gentle Cures: Safe and Effective Healing Therapies*. New York, New York: Sterling Publishing Co., Inc., 1997: 49.

[27] Ibid., 20.

[28] Tenney, Louise, M.H. *Health Handbook.* Pleasant Grove, Utah: Woodland Books, 1994: 189.

[29] Ibid., 164.

[30] Ibid., 164.

[31] Tenney, Louise, M.H. *The Encyclopedia of Natural Remedies.* Pleasant Grove, Utah: Woodland Publishing, Inc., 1995: 195.

[32] Tenney, Louise, M.H. *Health Handbook.* Pleasant Grove, Utah: Woodland Books, 1994: 196.

[33] Ibid., 197.

[34] Ibid., 201.

[35] Ibid., 201.

[36] Tenney, Louise, M.H. *The Encyclopedia of Natural Remedies.* Pleasant Grove, Utah: Woodland Publishing, Inc., 1995: 29.

[37] Ibid., 29.

[38] Moore, Michael *Herbs for the Urinary Tract: Herbal relief for kidney stones, bladder infections and other problems of the urinary tract.* New Canaan, Connecticut: Keats Publishing, Inc., 1998: 47.

[39] Tenney, Louise, M.H. *Health Handbook.* Pleasant Grove, Utah: Woodland Books, 1994: 147.

[40] Tierra, Lesley, L.Ac. *Herbalist The Herbs of Life: Health & Healing Using Western & Chinese Techniques.* Freedom, California: The Crossing Press, 1992: 65.

[41] Tenney, Louise, M.H. *Health Handbook.* Pleasant Grove, Utah: Woodland Books, 1994: 178.

[42] Ibid., 176.

[43] Castleman, Michael *The Healing Herbs: The Ultimate Guide to the Curative Power of Nature's Medicines.* New York: Bantam Books, 1991: 262.

[44] Tenney, Louise, M.H. *Health Handbook.* Pleasant Grove, Utah: Woodland Books, 1994: 176.

[45] Ibid., 168.

[46] Williams, Jude C., MH, ND *Nature's Gentle Cures: Safe and Effective Healing Therapies.* New York, New York: Sterling Publishing Co., Inc., 1997: 113.

[47] Ibid., 74.

48 Tenney, Louise, M.H. *Health Handbook*. Pleasant Grove, Utah: Woodland Books, 1994: 169.
49 Williams, Jude C., MH, ND *Nature's Gentle Cures: Safe and Effective Healing Therapies*. New York, New York: Sterling Publishing Co., Inc., 1997: 28.
50 Tenney, Louise, M.H. *Health Handbook*. Pleasant Grove, Utah: Woodland Books, 1994: 204.
51 Ibid., 192.
52 Ibid., 192.

Endnotes for Section 5

1 Tenney, Louise, M.H. *The Encyclopedia of Natural Remedies*. Pleasant Grove, Utah: Woodland Publishing, Inc., 1995: 302.
2 Ibid., 177.
3 Ibid., 259.
4 Tenney, Louise, M.H. *Health Handbook*. Pleasant Grove, Utah: Woodland Books, 1994: 29, 34.
5 Atkins, Robert C. *Dr. Atkins' Vita-Nutrient Solution: Nature's Answer to Drugs*. New York, New York: Simon & Schuster, 1999: 298.
6 Ibid., 299.
7 Ibid., 198.
8 Ibid., 198.
9 Tenney, Louise, M.H. *The Encyclopedia of Natural Remedies*. Pleasant Grove, Utah: Woodland Publishing, Inc., 1995: 193.
10 Atkins, Robert C. *Dr. Atkins' Vita-Nutrient Solution: Nature's Answer to Drugs*. New York, New York: Simon & Schuster, 1999: 272.
11 Tenney, Louise, M.H. *Health Handbook*. Pleasant Grove, Utah: Woodland Books, 1994: 91.
12 Ibid., 253-4.
13 Tenney, Louise, M.H. *The Encyclopedia of Natural Remedies*. Pleasant Grove, Utah: Woodland Publishing, Inc., 1995: 262.

References for "Vitamin and Minerals and IC"
Atkins, Robert C. *Dr. Atkins' Vita-Nutrient Solution: Nature's Answer to Drugs*. New York, New York: Simon & Schuster, 1999: 54-5, 57, 63, 70-1, 74-5, 77, 118, 122.

Krohn, Jacqueline, MD, Taylor, Frances A., MA, and Proseer, Jinger, LMT. *The Whole Way to Natural Detoxification: The complete guide to clearing your body of toxins.* Hartley & Marks Publishers, 1996: 135-6, 141.

Tenney, Louise, M.H. *Health Handbook.* Pleasant Grove, Utah: Woodland Books, 1994: 110-1, 125, 237, 265-9, 271, 278, 295.

Tenney, Louise, M.H. *The Encyclopedia of Natural Remedies.* Pleasant Grove, Utah: Woodland Publishing, Inc., 1995: 108, 147, 232-6, 259, 262, 280, 288, 302, 304, 329, 332, 388.

Other References

Borsaak, H. *Vitamins: What They Are and How They Can Effect You.* New York, U.S.A.: Pyramid Books, 1971.

Carter, Mildred and Weber, Tammy *Body Reflexology: Healing at Your Fingertips.* West Nyack, New York: Parker Publishing Company, 1994.

Houston, F.M., D.C. *The Healing Benefits of Acupressure: Acupuncture Without Needles.* New Canaan, Connecticut: Keats Publishing, Inc., 1991.

Rodenberg, H. and Feldzaman, A.N. *Doctors Book for Vitamin Therapy: Megavitamins for Health.* New York, U.S.A., 1974.

Ziff, S. *Silver Dental Fillings: The Toxic Timebomb.* Santa Fe, New Mexico, U.S.A.: Avery Publishing Group, 1985.

Appendix

Though it is nearly identical to the one in Dr. William Crook's book *The Yeast Connection* (which I would highly recommend, by the way), this candida quiz was taken (and very slightly modified) from The Yeast Answer Booklet from the Candida Wellness Center in Provo, Utah. If you would like more information on their anti-candida program or would like to read the entire booklet (which by the way is free and I think extremely helpful), you can call the Wellness Center at 1-800-869-1613. Keep in mind that the products they sell are somewhat expensive, but you don't have to buy the products to get the booklet and you don't have to buy ALL the products even if you want to try their program. Back when I did their anti-candida program, they didn't have near the amount of products they have now, so I'm not much help in that regard. But I can tell you that this is the place where I purchased colloidal silver and I did find it to be safe and effective. (Naturally this is just my opinion and should only be taken as such.) I offer the above information only because I am asked about it so often.

Candida Questionnaire

This questionnaire is designed for adults and the scoring system is not appropriate for children. It lists factors in your medical history, which promote the growth of the common yeast candida albicans (section A) and symptoms commonly found in individuals with yeast-connected illness (sections B and C).

On a separate piece of paper keep track of your score for each of the three sections. For each "yes" answer in section A, score the points after the corresponding question. Total your score for section A. Then move on to Sections B and C and score as directed.

Filling out and scoring this questionnaire should help you and your physician evaluate the possible role of yeasts in contributing to your health problems. Yet it will not provide an automatic "yes" or "no" answer.

Section A: History

1. Have you taken tetracycline or other antibiotics for acne for 1 month or longer? Score: 35 points

2. Have you at any time in your life, taken other "broad spectrum" antibiotics for respiratory, urinary, or other infections (for 2 months or longer or in shorter courses 4 or more times in a one year period?
    Score: 35 points

3. Have you taken a broad spectrum antibiotic even a single course?
    Score: 6 points

4. Have you at any time in your life been bothered by persistent prostatitis, vaginitis, or other problems affecting your reproductive organs?   Score: 25 points

5. Have you been pregnant...
2 or more times?	Score: 5 points
One time?	Score: 3 points

6. Have you taken birth control pills...
For more than 2 years?	Score: 15 points
For 6 months to 2 years?	Score: 8 points

7. Have you taken prednisone, decadron, or other cortisone-type drugs...
For more than 2 weeks?	Score: 15 points
For 2 weeks or less?	Score: 6 points

8. Does exposure to perfumes, insecticides, fabric shop odors, or other chemicals provoke...
Moderate to severe symptoms?	Score: 20 points
✓ Mild symptoms?	Score: 5 points

9. Are your symptoms worse on damp, muggy days or in moldy places?   Score: 20 points

10. Have you had athlete's foot, ring worm, "jock itch" or other chronic fungous infections of the skin or nails? Have such infections been...
Severe or persistent?	Score: 20 points
✓ Mild to moderate?	Score: 10 points

11. Do you crave sugar?   Score: 10 points

12. Do you crave breads?   Score: 10 points

13. Do you crave alcoholic beverages?   Score: 10 points

14. Does tobacco smoke *really* bother you? Score: 10 points

Total Score, Section A...51......

180

Section B: Major Symptoms

For each symptom present, mark the appropriate score on a separate piece of paper and then add together for a total score for section B.

If a symptom is occasional or mild score 3 points
If a symptom is frequent and/or moderately severe score 6 points
If a symptoms is severe and/or disabling score 9 points

1. Fatigue or lethargy *3*
2. Feeling of being "drained" *3*
3. Poor memory *6*
4. Feeling "spacey" or "unreal" *3*
5. Inability to make decisions *3*
6. Numbness, burning or tingling
7. Insomnia *9*
8. Muscle aches *3*
9. Muscle weakness or paralysis
10. Pain and/or swelling in joints *3*
11. Abdominal pain *3 Lower*
12. Constipation
13. Diarrhea *3*
14. Bloating, belching, or intestinal gas *3*
15. Troublesome vaginal burning, itching or discharge *6*
16. Prostatitis
17. Impotence
18. Loss of sexual desire *3*
19. Endometriosis or infertility *3*
20. Cramps and/or other menstrual irregularities
21. Premenstrual tension
22. Attacks of anxiety or crying *6 oNly recently*
23. Cold hands or feet and/or chilliness
24. Shaking or irritable when hungry

Total score, Section B......*60*..........................

Section C: Other symptoms
While the symptoms in this section occur commonly in patients with yeast-connected illness, they also occur commonly in patients who do not have candida.

For each symptom present, mark the appropriate score on a separate piece of paper and then add together for a total score for section C.

If a symptom is occasional or mild score 1 point
If a symptom is frequent and/or moderately severe score 2 points
If a symptom is severe and/or persistent score 3 points

1. Drowsiness 1
2. Irritability or jitteriness 2
3. Uncoordinated 2 Drop a lot of things
4. Inability to concentrate 2
5. Frequent mood swings 2 only recently
6. Headache 1
7. Dizziness/loss of balance 1
8. Pressure above ears...feeling of head swelling
9. Tendency to bruise easily 2
10. Chronic rashes or itching
11. Psoriasis or recurrent hives
12. Indigestion or heartburn 2
13. Food sensitivity or intolerance 2 esp. Now
14. Mucus in stools
15. Rectal itching
16. Dry mouth or throat 1
17. Rash or blisters in mouth 1½ canker sores, sml "blisters"
18. Bad breath 1
19. Foot, hair, or body odor not relieved by washing 2 Esp. Now
20. Nasal congestion or post nasal drip 1
21. Nasal itching
22. Sore throat 1
23. Laryngitis, loss of voice
24. Cough or recurrent bronchitis 1 Mornings esp

Section C: Other Symptoms (Continued)

25. Pain or tightness in chest
26. Wheezing or shortness of breath
27. Urinary frequency, urgency, or incontinence _3_
28. Burning on urination
29. Spots in front of eyes or erratic vision
30. Burning or tearing of eyes _2_
31. Recurrent infections or fluid in ears
32. Ear pain or deafness

Total score of Section C.........51.............................
Total score of Section B.......60.........................
Total score of Section A........31.............................

Grand Total Score from all 3 sections......142.........

The grand total score will help you and your physician decide if your health problems are yeast-connected. Scores in women will run higher as 7 items in the questionnaire apply exclusively to women, while only 2 apply exclusively to men.

Yeast-connected health problems are almost certainly present in women with scores over 180 and in men with scores over 140.
Yeast-connected health problems are probably present in women with scores over 120 and in men with scores over 90.
Yeast-connected health problems are possibly present in women with scores over 60 and in men with scores over 40.
With scores of less than 60 in women and 40 in men, yeasts are less apt to cause health problems.

Other books by Catherine M. Simone

To Wake In Tears
Understanding Interstitial Cystitis

Copyright © 1998
ISBN: 0-9667750-0-7

&

Awakening Through the Tears
Interstitial Cystitis and
the Mind/Body/Spirit Connection

Copyright © 2002
ISBN: 0-9667750-2-3

For more information, please visit http://www.ic-hope.com